jump for joy!

jump for joy!

BY ROY ALD

PUBLISHED BY

BERNARD GEIS ASSOCIATES

Acknowledgment is gratefully made to The New American Library for permission to quote from *Office Hours: Day and Night* by Janet Travell, M.D. © 1968.

CONTENTS

A NOTE FROM THE AUTHOR

I SHOULD LIKE to make clear the objectives of this book and how to use it to derive its real benefits.

Jump-rope exercise is intended to promote physical fitness as preventive therapy for the healthy person. Where exercise is to be prescribed for ailments already present—such as certain cardiovascular conditions, hypertension, respiratory and psychosomatic ills and so on—the only proper consultant is a physician. Our purpose is to prevent the onset of these and other ailments and to *raise* the general level of robust good health. The improvement in outlook and performance through a more vital energy exchange is equally important. And the desire for a more attractive, more youthful appearance should never be minimized.

This book is designed to help the reader recognize the effect of his personal lifestyle and activities upon general health, body weight, mental attitudes, virility and youthfulness. But, above all, it is a *perform-*

ance book. And the fitness activity it recommends is both easy to do—and *fun*. This fact is mentioned not as a form of sugar-coating: the title, *Jump for Joy!*, has been deliberately chosen because *enjoyment* is quite literally the key to its special effectiveness, for fun has a direct effect upon the body's internal chemistry as the activator of the vital organs. Without enjoyment, physical exertion cannot be truly *re-creational*, a medical fact that will be explained in common-sense language.

There are those readers who will want to go through every chapter, every section and chart, in sequence and in some detail. Others, more impatient, will want to take up a jump rope and begin the exercise instructions and then, perhaps, dip into other sections as their interest is captured. All of this is quite permissible, and allowances for such individual approaches are taken into account.

Some will have in mind goals of advanced physical conditioning, enabling them to participate in vigorous sports. Others will be pleased to keep themselves flexible and free of aches. A great many will be more interested in an attractive and trim appearance. *The Jump-Rope Exercise System* offers three graduated levels of activity. It is arranged to serve each person in his own way. And by utilizing the special section included for that purpose—*The Jump-rope Personalizer* section—it can be "customized" in even greater detail.

There is, however, one rule that *cannot* be breached. It is our "funmaker" approach. The reader will discover that pleasurable participation is emphasized in *all* jump-rope exercise sessions—standard, intermediate and advanced. It has determined the arrangement of the book so that you need never consider your exercising a chore at any time. For this reason, there is a complete *Funmaker Fitness* section; its purpose is to encourage the development of casual, playful jump-rope activities—for housewives filling idle moments while watching daytime television; for corporate personnel; secretaries; business and advertising brainstormers; and as a stimulus for ideas and a diversion from those over-caloried coffee breaks we all take. There are jump-rope games and contests for on- and off-campus fun, outings, and jet-set parties—sense and even some nonsense, to remind you that *fun and fitness* mix very well indeed.

iNTRodUcTioN

WHILE I PRESENT the *Jump-Rope Exercise System* as a personal triumph, I must confess that I can hardly claim it as an intentional development. As a physical-fitness professional who has conducted thousands of classes and groups over the years, I went from one exercise system to another in search of one that could effectively promote and maintain body health and fitness. Along the way, I persuaded myself—a common mistake of the profession—that it was not the exercises that were lacking but the *exercisers*. It seemed all too evident that they did not perform the exercises properly, with sufficient regularity or keep to an exercise program long enough before dropping out.

Whether prescribing calisthenics, isometrics, jogging, cycling, weight-lifting or various types of conditioning equipment, my experience was correspondingly disappointing. And I conducted groups as different as that of grade-school-age children and senior citizens, suburban housewives and clubwomen and executive and secretarial corporate personnel. The common response was waning enthusiasm, expressions of physical ordeal and gradually reduced efforts. Even among those with the greatest initial zeal, temporary gains were soon lost by frequent absences from exercise sessions. This on-again –off-again treadmill approach is identical to the pattern of the reducing dieter; and research on all diets over the past thirty-five years has proved them to be failures—even those including the weight-control groups.[1]

The fact that new exercise systems *and* diets, and combined versions of both, continue to proliferate is evidence of a public need that has not satisfactorily been met. My physical-fitness books—one on a calisthenic-exercise system, another on bicycling and a third on jogging—have all been part of my earnest effort to meet this need with a single effective exercise program that people would not only take up but stay with lastingly. And do so on their own, for the sheer pleasure of the physical invigoration.

Actually, one truly vigorous exercise *did* evoke this response from *all* of the individuals in the many different groups with which I had experience. I am referring to jump-rope activity. I kept jump ropes around and made them available as a way of a beneficial diversion. But to be perfectly frank, I resented the tendency of exercisers to drift away from the "real business" of each fitness session to engage in what I then regarded as a form of pleasant avoidance.

Apparently, the too obvious has a way of be-

[1] Stunkard, A. J., and M. McLaren-Hume, "The Results of Treatment for Obesity," *AMA Archives of Internal Medicine*, vol. 103 (1959), pp. 79–85.

ing overlooked. And I don't know why I or any other physical-fitness expert did not seize upon this universal fascination with jump-rope activity as a readily accessible solution, especially since the values of the exercise are well-known. For example, it is commonly used as an accompanying exercise in the physical-conditioning programs of even the most highly disciplined professional athletes. But eventually, more in the way of despair at not finding the effects I sought in other exercise programs, I focused my complete attention upon ropejumping— not as an accompanying exercise, *but rather as the basis for a complete physical-fitness program.*

It qualified in every respect: as a vigorous and deeply beneficial physical activity for the internal organs and the circulatory system, as well as for the entire musculo-skeletal frame. But of its effectiveness for other less obvious, though not less important, reasons, I did not become immediately aware. These uniformly positive benefits of jump-rope activity were revealed to me only through continued performance by countless exercisers.

I can hardly convey to the reader—and it is a delightful, exhilarating experience he will presently discover for himself—the transformation that took place in those exercise groups I subsequently conducted. The entire atmosphere changed from the familiar accompaniment of labored groans to one of joyful release. Individuals who really needed exercise and who were participating fully in deeply demanding physical exertions were suddenly "having fun." They needed no countdown, no childish coaxing or drill-master vigilance. More than that, it became obvious that with their rapid mastery of the various jump-rope skills, they were adopting the practice on their own, *away* from the group exercise sessions. Many began devising their own jump-rope exercises, and a goodly number of the exercises included in this book are adaptations of these personally created versions.

It soon became clear to me that ropejumping was that long-sought-after panacea for physical unfitness. At the same time, I recognized that it was strictly *bad news* for those interested in profiting from the "exercise industry," because ropejumping was essentially so simple, natural and enjoyable that it required no supervision. Further—as the reader will observe for himself after becoming acquainted with the basic instructions—no special time or place in terms of his attendance at a professional establishment is called for. Quite the contrary, ropejumping as an activity can easily be designed to suit the individual's lifestyle. In other words, physical exercise need no longer be an afterthought, saved up for the end of the day or crammed into the hurried moments of a sleepy-eyed morning in the way of a "treatment."

Happily and most beneficially, jumping rope permits the individual to *integrate* physical exercise into those special activity patterns that are his own. And instead of having to take one's "exercise dose," the approach becomes a positive one, a matter more fully explained in the material that follows. One could step out from behind a desk to take up a jump rope. Or while in the kitchen preparing meals. Or during TV commercials. And for so many reasons: to stimulate the circulation; to flex a stiff back or legs; to relax general tension in the neck and behind the eyes where headaches often begin; to clear the head and trigger mental alertness with increased oxygen flow for the brain; for a quickly revived, wide-awake appearance and a more efficient performance before an important business or social engagement. All of these and many other effects that promote enduring health and prolonged youthfulness are among the rewards of this extraordinary exercise.

"Physical fitness programs, good and bad, were the mode. For exercise, when I had been sitting too long in my office, I could have relied on simply jogging in place beside my desk, but it was more fun to jump rope. Scientific study had demonstrated that five minutes of rope skipping a day improved the physical condition of untrained subjects within a relatively short period. I kept several jump ropes handy and my nurse, my secretary, and I were known to have shut the doors and taken turns skipping rope in my inside treatment room.

The long, carpeted hall outside my door would have been a temptation to any rope-skipper. One evening when all was still, to the amusement of the White House guard, I turned my rope and jumped it at a run down the hall's length. Just as I started back from the far end of the soft red carpet, Caroline, John, and Miss Shaw entered unexpectedly after a late outing. I was caught. Caroline ran alongside me with envy and delight. Afterward, she would rush up to me at embarrassing moments and request loudly: 'Dr. Travell, please, I want to see you jump rope down the hall again.' "

—Janet Travell, M.D.
White House Physician
to President John F. Kennedy

PART I THE TEMPO of
HEALTH AND fitness

CHAPTER 1 **THE RHYTHMS of THE body**

THERE ARE MANY body rhythms. Science refers to them as "bio-rhythms," from "bio," meaning life. We are all familiar with the rhythms of heartbeat and pulse; of the digestion; of the replacement of old cells with new ones; of the menstrual and reproductive cycles; and even with the day-and-night rhythms to which we are attuned in sleep and waking. In fact, medical science has discovered that rapid jet travel across time zones can temporarily disturb these and other body cycles. Science has also shown that our brain rhythms show a pattern for each person as distinctive as his thumb print!

In infancy, the child uses his inborn rhythms to adapt to the outside world. If his rhythms are disordered, he may show the effects all of his life. Stammering and various speech defects point to a rhythmic upset of the nervous system. On this subject, the internationally renowned Professor René

Dubos of Rockefeller University has written: "Man, having evolved under the cosmic forces, has been 'imprinted' by the rhythms of nature—from those of the mother's heartbeat to those associated with the daily and seasonal cycles." [2]

In theory, a situation that is completely fulfilling all of the time would keep us rolling along, perfectly synchronized. It would make a perfectly balanced demand upon our human stuff. Our bodies do a remarkably good job of it, really, though the king-size share of the credit must go to these very same body rhythms. Nature wisely designed them as automatic timers. They work to keep the life cycles in balance—our body temperature, our blood composition, and others we have mentioned. However, these wonderful rhythms are not entirely self-regulating and foolproof. We can act upon them to keep them steady—or tilt them mildly, even seriously, out of vital balance. Physical activity figures prominently in this picture. And the *jump-rope exercise system* places an important instrument in your control to help maintain healthy body rhythms.

[2] René Dubos, "Environmental Determinants of Human Life," *Environmental Influences,* ed. David C. Glass (New York: The Rockefeller University Press and Russell Sage Foundation, 1968), p. 148.

tHε joyful
RhytHMs of hεΛlth

WHEN OVERCOME WITH buoyant feelings, we literally
jump for joy. Or we would, as readily as a child does,
if we had not been slowly drained of our natural
ebullience.

Since much of importance will be made of this
joie de vivre quality of ropejumping, an explanation is called for. First, it is necessary to point out
that every single human response derives from our
feelings, as confirmed research in the neurosciences
informs us.[3]

Our feelings are used by nature to signal us to
attend to the thousands of bodily functions that keep

---

[3] "Feelings stem from the most primordial and most
central nervous mechanisms. . . . Feeling states constitute
our original and most intimate experience. Everything
else we perceive is adventitious to feeling our existence."

Gardner C. Quarton (ed.) *et al., The Neurosciences*
(New York: The Rockefeller University Press, 1967).

us alive and healthy. We experience them as desires, cravings. It is these E-MOTIONS that excite us to MOTION, bringing into play our physical frame —muscles, joints, limbs and torso. A simple picture of the way it works is this: our glands secrete hormones, which is a word from the Greek, meaning "to excite." These hormones enter our bloodstream, and it is to the degree that they produce excitement in us that the heart, lungs, diaphragm —all of our *vital organs* in fact—set up the tempo of the body rhythms. We are most familiar with one of these hormonal *rhythm regulators* in the form of the pulse or heartbeat. In this case, the vital organs involved power the system with oxygen and MOTIVATE the frame muscles for physical action. When we speak of our *feelings* from now on, we can visualize them as the rhythm regulators of the vital organs and the pacesetters of physical action. And we can recognize the body's sequence for action as: E-MOTION = MOTIVATION = MOTION.

Now, for the special distinction that the body makes between *good* and *bad* feelings. When our nerve impulses reach the central nervous system in an *unrhythmic* way, they produce feelings of discomfort according to a degree of pain. *Pleasure* is associated with regular or harmonious rhythms. It is clear from this that reference to enjoyment, in any discussion of physical fitness, is of major importance and why it is a fundamental of the *Jump for Joy!* exercise system.

fatigue: sign of
disordered bio-rhythms

WITH THE INCREASING pronouncements of the President's Council on Physical Fitness and many reputable physicians, more people are becoming convinced of the importance of exercise. They have a high regard for the benefits spelled out in terms of improved health, fuller energy resources and a more youthful appearance. Many make resolutions to begin programs of regular exercise but somehow put off getting started. Others make a beginning that tapers off too soon and leaves them again with little more than their honest intentions.

One explanation for the neglect of a regular schedule of physical exercise is more common than all the rest. This excuse—the lack of time—is easily discounted by pointing out that some exercise schedules require no more than ten or fifteen minutes daily. No, it isn't really the time, although it is a common complaint of the housewife, business executive, secretary, or television performer, for that matter. "Just plain tiredness" or "weariness" or "exhaustion" . . . a lot of ways of saying the same thing, and they are all shades of the same medical term: *fatigue.*

The mistake is that such responses are casually brushed off. They should not be. The housewife with her own car and helpful household appliances and many free hours can feel terribly dragged out at the end of the day. The same for the office worker who pushes himself from his chair for brief periods a few times during the day. And yet, at the end of the day it becomes a real effort for him to make it home, where he then parks himself on the couch for the remainder of the evening in a state of exhaustion. For others, involved in business appointments or even cocktail partying, *despite the notable absence of any real physical exertion,* the tiredness of which they complain is very real.

"Fatigue has become," in the words of Dr. David McKrioch, Walter Reed Army Institute of Research, Washington, D.C., "the socially acceptable excuse for not doing things." So universal and uniquely common to our times is the phenomenon that medical science has applied itself to a careful study of its characteristics.

There are two major types:

Physiological Fatigue: it is the exhaustion that comes from heavy physical effort and drains the available energy of healthy muscles. Sound sleep was, and still remains, the proper prescription. It might be called *natural* fatigue. But it is the other kind that is the source of the difficulty of these persons already described.

Psychological Fatigue: it frequently comes from boredom, nervous tension and emotional upset. Whatever the reason, it will have this in common: an exceedingly low level of physical activity.

A study of some three hundred "fatigue" patients in Boston produced results in agreement with the broad general research on the subject. As high a figure as 80 percent of these people were found to be suffering from *psychological* fatigue.

This new type of fatigue is a product of our modern, largely mechanized way of life. Dr. Raymond D. Adams, Boullard Professor of Neuropathology, Harvard Medical School, has reported that this fatigue produces unique chemical changes in the body. The difference is that *rest or sleep does not recover the energies of the unphysically-spent group.*

The Harvard Fatigue Laboratory came to the conclusion that people so afflicted really needed a larger workload, providing a balanced coordination of muscular movements with deeper breathing and more active circulation.

Again, that medical sage of our nation, Dr. Paul Dudley White, has a pertinent word on the subject: "For optimal function of an alert brain, a really good blood supply is needed—and this means not only avoidance of over-nutrition, but also physical fitness in terms of firm and active muscles."

This opinion is seconded by another medical expert on the subject of fatigue, Dr. Hugh O. Thompson. He plainly states that "rest is not the proper treatment." He is another advocate of brisk exercise.

An impressive line-up of authorities lastingly

emphasizes this point for us: *the lack of physical exertion weakens the bio-rhythms, sapping the life energy and the motivation or* will *to exercise.*

It is an unhappy treadmill. Once you are on it, it continues to reduce physical capacity and exaggerate the feeling of exhaustion until the result is *chronic* fatigue. This is another medical term. It is a condition in which the vital body rhythms are at a really low ebb, and they stay there.

bio-rHyThmic exercise:

THE GREAT RESTORER

WILL ANY KIND of exercise serve the purpose of reducing fatigue? No. And it is important to know why, so that it is possible, once and for all, to step off the disappointing treadmill of new exercise systems as they are offered in what has become the "physical-fitness marketplace." And, in a more positive sense, it is essential to know what kind of exercise to concentrate on and how to apply it to one's personal needs.

To cut through a great deal of the advertising jargon used by any of hundreds of exercise systems, professionally speaking these systems fall into these three classifications:

- *Aerobic,* or oxygen-intake, exercises dealing with the vital-organ system.
- *Isometric,* or muscle-stress, exercises for the body frame with little body movement.

- *Isotonic,* or muscle and body movement, exercises in the calisthenic and gymnastic sense. These are also principally outer- or body-frame developers.

Any exercise system that does not take into account the body as a balanced bio-rhythmic whole is acting against nature's own design. For exercise to give significant benefits, it should exercise body function as nature intended. Overemphasis on one part of the body limits the benefits and, in some instances, can even be damaging to the person who suffers from hypertension and undertakes isometric or muscle-stress exercises, for example. And those hurried and harried people who engage in rapid calisthenic sessions are certainly not doing themselves any good.

Often the effectiveness of many sound exercise systems, especially those of the aerobic variety, is sacrificed for reasons that *seem* quite trivial. For instance, jogging can be wonderful exercise, and so can bicycling. Yet, my experience has shown me that many people find such exercise unsuitable and give up on it. And I am not about to classify as *trivial* any factor that results in the termination of exercise. Among the most common of these: restrictions on performance ranging from inconvenience, inclemency of the weather for outdoor exercise,[4] embarrassment at participation in an activity with which one is not comfortable, complaints of "not being good at it" or simply "hating every minute of it."

[4] As for *indoor* "stationary" jogging or cycling, the substitution is poor and joyless. There is a notable difference, as well, in the mechanics of bodily exertion.

By now, the reader is aware of the implications of trying to impose a disagreeable (for whatever reason!) physical-fitness program on the underexercised person. His vital rhythms are sluggish and so his motivation is definitely down. The activation he needs should be both re-creational and *enjoyable* to stimulate vital rhythm activators. To place upon the underexercised person the burden of having to drive himself into physical activity that he *abhors* is worthless. Such exercise regimens cannot be maintained for long.

CHAPTER 5 jump Rope: The ideal Rhythm exercise

THE CHOICE OF A physical activity that is familiar as a child's game confirms the bio-rhythmic needs it satisfies. For the child, it is a naturally joyous expression of the inborn body rhythms. It is an extension of that same performance we observe in the infant's early hand-held "dancing" response to music. Everyone *can* jump rope. The activity automatically evokes smiles, and its playful participation has a ready contagion. It can be performed easily and conveniently in many places and at many times. And the activity can easily be personalized according to an individual's age and physical condition and can be designed for a progressive build-up and revitalization of the natural body rhythms.

The jump-rope activity vigorously exercises the vital-organ regulators and the muscle frame. In its stimulation of the heart, lungs, diaphragm, the entire cardiovascular system, it is powerfully aerobic.

- Dr. Paul Dudley White reminds us of the physiological and psychological benefits of circulatory excercise. "Blood-clot prevention and the delaying of serious arterial sclerosis affecting heart, brain and kidneys are clear-cut results of this essential health regimen which needs to be emphasized far and wide in this era of our slavery to machines of all kinds." The vigorous use of the legs acts as a circulation booster, relieving the heart of 30 percent of its load.
- The studies of the Metropolitan Life Insurance Company have led it to recommend circulatory exercise to aid in the reduction of the fatty substances in the blood known as cholesterol.
- Circulatory exercises ward off the disease of the joints associated with aging.
- Such deep-down exercises improve the tone of the digestive system.
- They prolong reproductive vigor and youthfulness.
- The fuller oxygen intake aids the internal muscles in their operation of the vital organs.

The jumping effect uses the body weight, rhythmically raised from the ground and "caught" with a rigorous exercise of the bones, joints, connective tissue and muscles. In this respect, it is both isometric and isotonic. This means stronger bone calcium, the development of additional vital red-blood cells and greater joint lubrication and flexibility. All are important to prevent the crippling diseases that afflict so great a cross section of our population. This includes all kinds of muscular aches, backache and arthritic bone and joint ailments.

And the center from which all of this emerges is—*feeling*, which is synonymous with life itself. As the tempo regulator for the natural body rhythms, it is the literal "heartbeat" for the vital organs, energizing the thinking processes as well as the body frame. Physical fitness, in this sense, is the fitness measure of being alive. This is the new, all-inclusive focus through which exercise must be pursued.

To *jump for joy* is a lesson from nature in the fullest exercise of the natural body rhythms. It is expressive of the life urge to "let go" and exert the deeper human potential. In the words of Thomas Carlyle,

> *Let each become all that*
> *he was created capable of being;*
> *expand, if possible, to his full growth;*
> *and show himself at length*
> *in his own shape and stature,*
> *be these what they may.*

PART II THE JUMP-ROPE EXERCISE SECTION

All about the jump-rope exercise

Enjoyment: the pleasure and play value of the jump-rope activity eliminates "exercise ordeal." It begins with nature's regulator of the bio-rhythms. It promotes the vital balance of physical and psychological benefits.

Bio-Rhythmic: ropejumping surpasses all other exercises in this category, which supports all life.

Energy Output: jumping rope burns up as many calories as running—800 to 1100 calories per hour. It exceeds that of bicycling and calisthenics by 200 to 500 calories.

Internal Stimulation: the jump-rope leaping and bounding movements are superior to bicycling and more complete than running in the fuller arm and upper-torso movements. Ropejumping is equally effective in the activation of the vital organs and the depth of respiration. (Few calisthenic exercises are deeply circulatory.)

Coordination: no more perfect unity of grace, timing and coordination is to be found in physical exercise.

Participation Range: jump-rope exercise qualifies for both the male and female frame and physiology. And for the widest span of age groups.

Scheduling Convenience: both running and bicycling, to be effective, require extremely large areas, preferably outdoors as recommended by the various physicians and physical educators. (Effectiveness drops drastically in stationary cycling and running in place.) Seasons and weather conditions present problems that do not exist in jump-rope exercise. The small time requirement and the suitability of virtually any space encourage ropejumping with frequent regularity.

Level of Physical Condition: jump-rope exercises offer wide latitude for graduating exertions, from low levels of physical conditioning to high standards of athletic proficiency.

CHAPTER 7

HEAdsTARTER:

the Ropeless jump-off

My own experience with so many people I have reintroduced to jump-rope activity has proved the usefulness of the following jump-off routines—to be performed *without* the use of the rope. I say "*reintroduced*" because practically everyone has jumped rope at one time or another, and even if no more recently than childhood, it is surprising how easily the skill can be revived. And the jump-off exercises without the rope have been designed to help make the reintroduction even easier and more enjoyable. But they have an additional purpose—actually *several*— that make their continued use advisable throughout the standard jump-rope exercise section and, for many, at the intermediate jump-rope exercise level as well.

For the jump-rope novice and those who have been away from *vigorous* exercise for a prolonged period, a ropeless jump-off is a sensible prescription. It loosens the joints, eases muscular tension and re-regulates breathing. The fact that this acts to restore harmonious body rhythms explains the continued usefulness of these jump-offs even for the more adept.

Restored coordination comes on quickly, and *this* is the secret for a smooth and effortless jump-rope exercise performance. A few minutes of such random jumping, and one slips more easily into tempo with the spin of the rope.

Even if no express instructions were given as to *how much* of such exercises to take before picking up the rope, the participant himself would *feel* it. The body quickly seeks its own tempo when any kind of rhythmic movements are undertaken, with the mind "playing off" little rhythmic cadences. Try it for yourself by attempting some finger-snapping beat *before* such jumping—and then *after*. It is like the improved sensitivity to musical rhythms that takes over after several minutes of dancing. And the combination of a rhythmic performance of *jump* movements promotes a genuine sense of exhilaration. The bounding, leaping action literally (even if for an instant) defies gravity and inspires a joyous release. The experience gives one an insight into the rationale behind the tribal "jump" dances all over the world.

Everything in our daily lives—from the clothes we wear, the restraint of our movements, the conventional scheduling of our activities—tends to keep us to a rather "soldierly" social performance. How good it is to suddenly let go! To leap up and fling out one's arms. The pleasantness of the sensation becomes immediately obvious in the easing lines of facial expression. Jumping is fun. And it should be done not with the consciousness of this or that objective, but simply to celebrate being truly *alive!* These ropeless jump-offs can be performed in any corner and at any given time, and they are ideal as jump-rope headstarters.

THE HEEL-LIFT JUMP

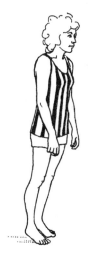

Hang loose, as if a harness were under your armpits, and lift yourself slightly so that your heels leave the ground with your toes barely touching. It is the mildest jumping action. It is prescribed for those who have been away a long time from jump-action exercise, with rusty joints and stiff tendons in need of a gradually increasing blood flow. And it is a must for senior citizens in good health who wish to get into jump-rope activity to maintain and elevate the level of their physical performance.

As in all of the other jump-off movements, the point is to keep it *rhythmic.*

- Maintain a moderate tempo.
- Perform the heel lift in 3 sets of 10 jumps each.
- Recover breathing between each set.
- Repeat from the beginning.

THE KNEE JUMP

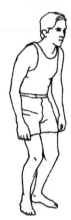

From a slight forward crouch—more of a stooping position—this rhythmic jump is made from a bend of the knee. The jumping effect is concentrated on the knees, the flexibility of which is of the utmost importance in ropejumping. It is a low jump.

- Maintain a moderate tempo.
- Perform the exercise in 3 sets of 10 jumps each.
- Recover breathing between each set.
- Repeat from the beginning.

THE SPACE JUMP-OFF

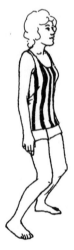

Perform this jump with both legs and with feet about 18 inches apart. The effect of the jump is to be felt in the inside and upper thighs and the vitals.

- Maintain a moderate tempo,
- Perform the exercise in 3 sets of 10 jumps each.
- Recover breathing between each set.
- Repeat from the beginning.

THE APACHE JUMP
A combination hop/jump, rhythmically alternating from left to right leg.

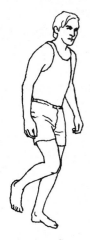

- Maintain a moderate tempo.
- Perform the exercise in 3 sets of 10 jumps each.
- Recover breathing between each set.
- Repeat from the beginning.

THE SOAR
An easy, upward, moderate-to-high leap that *must* be performed in a relaxed state. Smile. It may be a silly grin—but the all-over muscle relaxation is worth it.

- Begin with a moderate tempo and increase the rhythmic beat of each set.
- Perform the exercise in 3 sets of 10 jumps each.
- Recover breathing between each set.
- Repeat from the beginning.

THE FLING-
WING JUMP

Fling your arms high above your head, and then wide, horizontal to the shoulders. It must be in accord with each upward leap, as if in celebration. Of what? Why not celebrate *yourself* and that untapped capacity for joy inside you, waiting to be released!

- Maintain a moderate tempo.
- Perform the exercise in 3 sets of 10 jumps each.
- Recover breathing between each set.
- Repeat from the beginning.

SPECIAL
INSTRUC-
TIONS

For jump-rope novices who have been away from vigorous exercise: the ropeless jump sessions are suggested twice daily for one week or when the muscle or joint stiffness of the unaccustomed activity eases off, before taking up the jump rope.

For jump-rope novices who are more than mildly active: the jump-offs may be undertaken along with or prior to the jump-rope exercises. "More than *mildly active*" would mean that you are capable of walking for five minutes at a *vigorous* pace without excessive strain or hard breathing.

For senior citizens: the jump-offs are recommended on alternate days for four weeks before taking up the jump rope. THE SOAR exercise should be omitted, as well as any form of "high" jumps. The tempo adopted should be slow to moderate, but without any sacrifice of a rhythmic beat.

For the accomplished jumper: THE APACHE, THE SOAR and THE FLING-WING may be regularly used to advantage, at moderate to rapid step-up tempos, before taking up the jump rope for the most rhythmically coordinated effect.

CHAPTER 8 **ON THE MARK with jump-rope**

MANY READERS MAY BE of the opinion that, with a rope in hand, the only signal need be—GO! There is, however, more to the jump-rope exercise than meets the eye. It is true that anyone can do it. But there are a few principles, which, if mastered in the beginning, can help to:

- Make you more skillful and give you greater pleasure because of your increased skills.
- Prepare your system gradually for more intense jump-rope exercise.

SELECTING A JUMP ROPE

The Ball-Bearing Swivel Jump Rope: the spin occurs within the handle at the ball-bearing source.

The Spring-Swivel Jump Rope: it allows a free spin of the rope from the point of the swivel attachment hooked into the handle.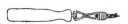

Five-and-Dime Model: with handles minus swivel and ball bearings. The spin is all in the jumper's wrist action.

The Old Clothesline: again, the spin is in the jumper's sleight of hand.

Yes, the jump ropes are superior in an ascending order. But it is possible to make do with any model if the rope has a fairly good *weight* to it and is of the proper length. About the rope itself, these days it is to be found in plastic, nylon, leather; by the time this book is published, I wouldn't be surprised at suede and mink jump ropes! But whatever the rope of *your* choice, try to keep in mind that it isn't what you have but how you use it!

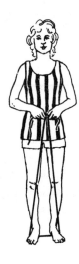

The Proper Length of the Jump Rope: assume a standing position with the feet parallel and spaced 3 or 4 inches apart. Trap the jump rope beneath both insteps. Now bring together the top ends of the rope (minus the handles). They should meet at, or close to, the point of the jumper's navel.

A Word About Jump-Rope Attire: you're pretty much on your own where this is concerned, but always: 1. loosen tie, collar, scarf, or anything constricting around the neck, the wrists, ankles or anywhere the circulation might be hampered; 2. wear the most comfortable footgear—preferably sneakers—or loosen shoelaces or, better still, remove shoes. High heels are out.

STARTING JUMP-ROPE POSITION

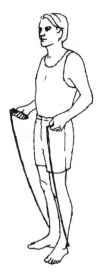

Stand with natural posture. Place your feet parallel, 3 or 4 inches apart for best balance. Put your arms at your sides and bent at the elbow, upraised to "driver position." The jump rope should be around the back of the ankles and drawn taut. Grasp the jump-rope handles in a "gun-holster" position. Hold the jump rope firmly but without tensing your hands.

The Basic Jump Turn: breaking slightly at the knees, bring weight forward, heels upraised, and make a slight jump. Timed simultaneously with the jump: the arms are dropped to gun-holster level and the rope spun over the head to pass beneath the feet in jump motion. *Keep the head up.* Do not look at the feet. *Do not observe the action of the rope.* Fix on an imaginary or real point ahead at eye level. *Concentrate upon the rhythm and the pleasant sensation of the jumping action.*

Now try it, just to prove to yourself that you can still do it. . . . All right, hold it. You're better than you thought. But remember, we do have our preliminaries, and if we go through this once, it will save a lot of frustration later on—no unnecessary stops and starts, rope-tripping, staggered rhythms, unconscious shifting of hand and foot positions and so on.

FOUR FOOT POSITIONS

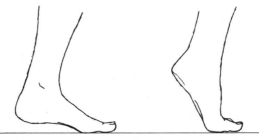

Ball-of-Foot or Forward Position. The most common.

Toe-Jump Position. The body weight forward and completely upon underside of toes. A more advanced position.

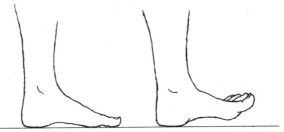

Flat-Foot Position. For special exercises only.

Heel-Jump Position. For special exercises only.

HAND POSITIONS

The arm-spin. The arms at driver position. The principal rope motion is created by the tossing of the arms in wide, inward circles. This is used frequently throughout to deliberately activate the upper torso while jumping. It also gives a relaxed and pleasant "free-style" sensation.

The hand-spin. The hands at holster level, creating the spin with hardly discernible wrist motions. For higher levels of jump/turn proficiency.

THE JUMP
STEPS

The two-step. A double jump for each single rope spin. The first jump is followed instantly by what is known as an "echo jump." It is more a rhythmic second beat. *The rope does not pass under the feet at the echo step.* The sequence is: spin-jump/touch, spin-jump/touch, spin-jump/touch.

The one-step. A single jump for each single rope spin.

The running-step. A single running step for each rope spin from a stationary position.

Try the movements to get the feel of these key jump steps:

> *Movement:* the two-step
> *Movement:* the one-step
> *Movement:* the running-step

JUMP-ROPE
TEMPOS

The rhythms to jump by are as important as any other feature in *The Jump-Rope Exercise System.* In this preliminary section, a simple device is used to help accustom you to: keeping a regular beat while jumping; and distinguish the three basic jump-rope tempos—SLOW/MEDIUM/FAST.

Our "metronome" will be that song of 1890 vintage, "Old MacDonald Had A Farm." It lends itself to a readily describable beat:

Slow	OLD	MAC	DON	ALD	HAD	A	FARM
	EEE	AIY	EEE	AIY	O		

Medium OLD-MAC-DON-ALD-HAD-A-FARM
EEE-AIY-EEE-AIY-O

Fast OLDMACDONALDHADAFARM
EEEAIYEEEAIYO

You will be able to practice tempo in the first jump-rope exercise movement: THE TRAIN. This is a warm-up exercise with which you will always begin each jump-rope session. Once the tempos become established in your mind, you will no longer need to think of the "Old MacDonald" refrain. In regular jump-rope sessions, this will be substituted by a count of the number of jump/ turns.

Practice Sequence:

Exercise	THE TRAIN
Special Focus	General warm-up. Restoring normal body rhythms.
Position	Basic jump-rope stance.
Action	Arm-spin, two-step. Begin *slow* tempo. Graduate to *medium* tempo. Accelerate to *fast* tempo. Try not to interrupt the flow.
Count	5 jump/turns—slow (Two-step) 10 jump/turns—medium (Two-step) 5 jump/turns—fast (One-step)

Rest

Repeat Sequence

CHAPTER 9

THE STANDARD

JUMP-ROPE EXERCISES

THE EXERCISES HAVE been given names that describe the movements. The reader will find that this will enable him to fix the exercise quickly and lastingly in his mind.

THE TRAIN   *See* page 41.

THE SAG   *Special Focus:* [5] Relaxation of joints and easing of nerve tension.

[5] All exercises are circulatory and general conditioners. The *Special Focus* pinpoints areas of the body activated with particular emphasis. This information is used in *Personalizing Jump-Rope Exercise*, page 134.

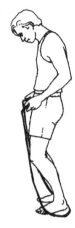

Position: Assume basic jump-rope stance. Breathe in and out slowly and deeply several times. Exhale and allow the body to sag, with head falling easily forward on chest, arms dangling, hands loose. Sag at knees.

Action: Jump with general body limpness. Allow head and limbs to "go their own way."

HOP 'N' JUMP   *Special Focus:* Thigh and buttock conditioner.

Position: Basic jump-rope stance.

Action: With alternate jump/turns, hop to oblique right and to oblique left.

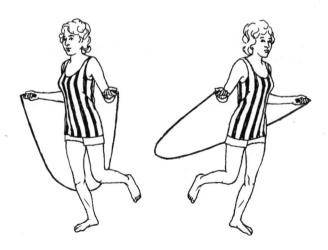

THE PRANCE

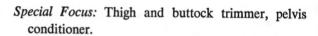

Special Focus: Thigh and buttock trimmer, pelvis conditioner.

Position: Basic jump stance.

Action: Stationary running jump with maximum knee lift, thigh at right angle to body, with toe pointed down.

THE GROUCHO

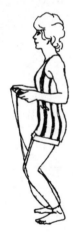

Special Focus: Conditions lower back and knee joints.

Position: Back straight, exaggerated bend at knees.

Action: Proceed to jump/turn while remaining in crouch position throughout the exercise.

THE PEACOCK

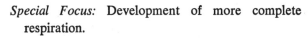

Special Focus: Development of more complete respiration.

Position: Stand erect, with exaggerated "West Point" stance—shoulder blades back, chest thrust out, inflated, head slightly upraised.

Action: Inhale and exhale deeply, alternating from THE SAG to THE PEACOCK during the regular jump action. Inhale PEACOCK/exhale SAG, inhale PEACOCK/exhale SAG.

THE
GREYHOUND

Special Focus: Build and strengthen abdominal muscle wall.

Position: Incline upper torso forward. Suck in stomach (this will be difficult in the beginning but will become surprisingly simple as control of the abdominal muscles is established).

Action: Follow regular jump/turn pattern while holding stomach in.

**THE
SWAYBACK**

Special Focus: To strengthen the tendons of the back and the spinal column.

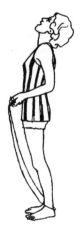

Position: Regular jump stance. With a slight bend at the knees, arch the back. Make as deep an inward curvature as possible.

Action: Hold to this position while doing a series of regular jump/turns.

**THE
STAR-SWALLOW**

Special Focus: Encourage firmer and more youthful jaw and neckline.

Position: From regular jump stance, raise and tilt head as far back as possible, stretching neck upward, with mouth wide open toward ceiling.

Action: While making regular jump/turns, alternately open and close mouth, stretching jaws wide as if to "swallow a star."

THE CHAPLIN

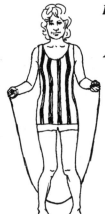

Special Focus: Benefit to inner thighs and pelvis, outer buttocks.

Position: Bend at knees. Assume a heel-to-heel foot position, with toes pointing out to sides.

Action: Retain this position during a series of regular jump/turns.

THE
PIGEON-TOE

Special Focus: Strengthens ankle and hip joints.

Position: Reverse of THE CHAPLIN. A toe-to-toe stance.

Action: Hold toe-to-toe position while performing regular jump/turns.

THE HIP
SWING—LEFT

Special Focus: Prevent stiffening of hip joints and lower spinal column.

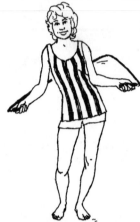

Position: From regular jump stance, break (displace) hip to the left.

Action: Hold to this position while performing regular jump/turns.

THE HIP
SWING—RIGHT

Repeat exercise with the hip displaced to the right side.

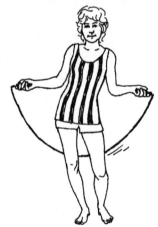

THE STIFF

Special Focus: A head-to-toe muscle contraction and joint conditioner.

Position: Stand erect. Tense all muscles; stiffen at joints.

Action: Maintain stiffness while performing regular jump/turns, with arms stiff. Rope-turn action in wrists only.

THE
MARATHON

Special Focus: Endurance. Break through to higher levels of internal and external body conditioning.

Position: Basic jump stance. Hand-spin, one-step.

Action: Smooth, relaxed motions; consistent *medium* tempo.

MASTERING
THE
STANDARD
JUMP-ROPE
EXERCISES

Your objectives in this section are to:

• Learn the exercise positions.
• Condition your body gradually for regular exercise sessions.
• Improve your jump-rope skills to the point that releases your natural rhythms.

Each orientation session will consist of four jump-rope exercises. Except for THE MARATHON, jump-rope exercises will be divided into 4 groups, with a jump-rope count of 10 for each. This will permit a rest between each group.

Example:

THE TRAIN

Full count: 40

10 jump/turns
    Rest

10 jump/turns
    Rest

10 jump/turns
  Rest

10 jump/turns
  Rest

The exercises of each orientation session will be considered mastered when the 4 groups (10 each) are completed with no more than two misses.

When a miss occurs, that group (10 count) is to begin again.

Repeat the same orientation exercise session until all of its exercises are mastered.

Rest means full breathing recovery. As your body becomes accustomed to the increasing activity, the rest period between exercise groups will be shortened. Breathing recovery will be more prompt.

DO NOT continue any orientation exercise session beyond a period of *5 minutes of actual jumping time,* exclusive of rest time.

DO NOT exercise for more than two complete sessions in any one day during the orientation period.

DO NOT move on to the next exercise until the preceding ones are mastered.

THE FUNMAKER APPROACH If you find yourself stymied during any single exercise session, if you are too impatient to perfect any exercise and if you are missing too often and having to start again, I recommend the Funmaker Approach.

1. Stop all attempts to complete the session according to the rules.

2. Take up the rope and just jump for the *fun* of it. Do THE TRAIN and THE MARATHON if you like, or neither one. Play with the movements—the two-step and one-step; the arm-spin and hand-spin; the ball-of-foot step, toe-jump step, flat-foot step. Do any jump-rope maneuver that comes to mind or one you do well. Fill in for the number of times you need to conclude the session.

3. Go to Part III, *Funmaker Fitness,* and have a ball.

4. Take up the regular session next time. And if it doesn't work out, go back to the *Funmaker* section. In time, it will work out. Do not stubbornly insist upon perfection too soon. Forcing the issue will only throw you out of rhythm and add to the difficulty. With the *Funmaker* approach, you are jumping and earning the benefit of circulatory exercise. And . . . you are improving your technique.

ORIENTA-
TION
SESSIONS

Two of the four exercises in each session (after the first) will be repeats. The exerciser is therefore expected to master two new positions within each session. THE TRAIN and THE MARATHON are the repeats. The first as warm-up, and to refine jump/turns, skills and rhythms. The second, THE MARATHON, is the incentive exercise to serve, as well, as an improvement measure. It is the only one of the four exercises with a varying count.

Unless otherwise noted, the exercises are to be performed in the *Two-step, Arm-spin, Ball-of-foot Position,* at *Medium Tempo.*

First Session	THE TRAIN	THE SAG	THE PEACOCK	THE MARATHON
	Count 10 Rest	Count 10 Rest	Count 10 Rest	Hand-spin/ one-step
	Count 10 Rest	Count 10 Rest	Count 10 Rest	Jump until
	Count 10 Rest	Count 10 Rest	Count 10 Rest	you miss
	Count 10 Rest	Count 10 Rest	Count 10 Rest	Maximum count: 50

Second Session	THE TRAIN	THE GREYHOUND	THE HOP 'N' JUMP	THE MARATHON
	Count 10 Rest	Count 10 Rest	Count 10 Rest	Hand-spin/ one-step
	Count 10 Rest	Count 10 Rest	Count 10 Rest	Jump until
	Count 10 Rest	Count 10 Rest	Count 10 Rest	you miss
	Count 10 Rest	Count 10 Rest	Count 10 Rest	Maximum count: 50

Third Session	THE TRAIN	THE PRANCE	THE GROUCHO	THE MARATHON
	Count 10 Rest	Count 10 Rest	Count 10 Rest	Hand-spin/ one-step
	Count 10 Rest	Count 10 Rest	Count 10 Rest	Jump until
	Count 10 Rest	Count 10 Rest	Count 10 Rest	you miss
	Count 10 Rest	Count 10 Rest	Count 10 Rest	Maximum count: 50

Fourth Session	THE TRAIN	THE SWAYBACK	THE STAR-SWALLOW	THE MARATHON
	Count 10 Rest	Count 10 Rest	Count 10 Rest	Hand-spin/ one-step
	Count 10 Rest	Count 10 Rest	Count 10 Rest	Jump until
	Count 10 Rest	Count 10 Rest	Count 10 Rest	you miss
	Count 10 Rest	Count 10 Rest	Count 10 Rest	Maximum count: 50

Fifth Session	THE TRAIN	THE CHAPLIN	THE PIGEON-TOE	THE MARATHON
	Count 10 Rest	Count 10 Rest	Count 10 Rest	Hand-spin/ one-step
	Count 10 Rest	Count 10 Rest	Count 10 Rest	Jump until
	Count 10 Rest	Count 10 Rest	Count 10 Rest	you miss
	Count 10 Rest	Count 10 Rest	Count 10 Rest	Maximum count: 50

Sixth Session	THE TRAIN	THE HIP SWING	THE STIFF	THE MARATHON
	Count 10 Rest	Count 10 Rest	Count 10 Rest	Hand-spin/ one-step
	Count 10 Rest	Count 10 Rest	Count 10 Rest	Jump until
	Count 10 Rest	Count 10 Rest	Count 10 Rest	you miss
	Count 10 Rest	Count 10 Rest	Count 10 Rest	Maximum count: 50

Some Useful Sidelights: Here are some interesting and useful details for you to consider as you begin your regular exercise sessions.

Jump-rope exercise equals 1000 calories per hour, which equals approximately 16½ calories per minute.

Eight minutes of jump-rope exercise (average jump-rope session) are equal to approximately 132 calories.

Remember here the importance of physical activity in balancing the energy scale. If you consider calories going out in the form of energy, you are most likely to be conscious of the amount of calories going in, in the form of food. (See *Your E.Q.* (*Energy Quotient*), page 113.)

Although each exercise session has an allotted time, the exerciser does not have to be distracted by keeping his eye on the clock. This chore has been eliminated by figuring out the number of jump/turns in set-time sequences.

Using the *medium tempo, two-step* there is an average of: *80 jump/turns per minute; 40 jump/turns per ½ minute; and 20 jump/turns per 15 seconds.*

Using the *medium tempo, one-step* there is an average of: *120 jump/turns per minute; 60 jump/turns per ½ minute; and 30 jump/turns per 15 seconds.*

You do not have to memorize any of this. The jump-rope count will be included with each exercise. This handy measure of jump/turns equated with time will come to register permanently as you go along.

REGULAR
WEEKLY
SCHEDULES

- *Minimum* number of jump-rope workouts: 6 per week, once daily. One rest day.
      Recommended: 12 per week, twice daily.
- Exercise Schedules A and B, which follow, are to be performed on alternate days.
- Unless otherwise noted, all exercises are to be performed at *medium tempo/ball-of-foot position/arm-spin position/two-step.*
- Continue with standard jump-rope exercise schedule a *minimum* of 8 successive weeks. Those satisfied with this level of activity may permanently continue it. Others may proceed to the intermediate level.

STANDARD
EXERCISE
SCHEDULE A

Energy Output Approximately 100+ Calories
This is a 10 minute exercise session.* But there is no need for clock-watching. All you need to do is to follow the count given with each exercise.

Warm-up   THE TRAIN

Count 10 slow (two-step)
Count 20 medium (one-step)
Count 10 fast (one-step)
  Rest
  Repeat

* With each exercise, unless otherwise noted, a count of 20 equals approximately 15 seconds. Rest equals the same interval. Each exercise is performed twice, for a total time per set equaling 1 minute.

Set 1	THE SAG	*Set 2*	THE PEACOCK

Set 1   THE SAG

Count 20
Rest
Count 20
Rest

Set 2   THE PEACOCK

Count 20
Rest
Count 20
Rest

Set 3   THE GREYHOUND

Count 20
Rest
Count 20
Rest

Set 4   THE HOP 'N' JUMP

Count 20
Rest
Count 20
Rest

Set 5   THE PRANCE

Count 20
Rest
Count 20
Rest

Set 6   THE GROUCHO

Count 20
Rest
Count 20
Rest

Set 8   THE STAR-SWALLOW

Set 7   THE SWAYBACK

Count 20
Rest
Count 20
Rest

THE STAR-SWALLOW

Count 20
Rest
Count 20
Rest

Endurance Jump   THE MARATHON

Continuous one-step.
Keep a record of each session.
Attempt to surpass previous sessions each
time to reach a maximum count of 200.

STANDARD   Energy Output
EXERCISE   Approximately 100+ Calories
SCHEDULE B   Same instructions as in Schedule A apply.

Warm-up   THE TRAIN

Count 10 slow (two-step)
Count 20 medium (two-step)
Count 10 fast (one-step)

Set 1	THE SAG	*Set 2*	THE PEACOCK
	Count 20		Count 20
	Rest		Rest
	Count 20		Count 20
	Rest		Rest
Set 3	THE GREYHOUND	*Set 4*	THE HOP 'N' JUMP
	Count 20		Count 20
	Rest		Rest
	Count 20		Count 20
	Rest		Rest
		Set 6	THE PIGEON-TOE
Set 5	THE CHAPLIN		
	Count 20		Count 20
	Rest		Rest
	Count 20		Count 20
	Rest		Rest
Set 7	THE HIP SWING	*Set 8*	THE STIFF
	Count 20		Count 20
	Rest		Rest
	Count 20		Count 20
	Rest		Rest

Endurance Jump

THE MARATHON

Continuous one-step.
Keep a record of each session.
Attempt to exceed your record each
time to reach a maximum count of 200.

tHE iNTERMEdiATE
JuMP-ROPE EXERCiSES

IF YOU HAVE followed the instructions of *The Jump-Rope Exercise System* and are reading beyond the standard schedules, then

- You have observed the improvement of your system from lower to increased activity quotas.
- You feel more fit and wish to advance to higher levels of fitness.
- You have established a 200 count in *The Marathon.*
- Your Pulse Test (See p. 68) has indicated your readiness for this progression.

A remarkable attribute of the human body is its ability to extend its performance. Each time, it graduates to a new plateau at which it levels off for awhile. There it undergoes a readjustment in balance, and the new and deeper rhythms take over. Your pulse recovery within the given time is evidence that you can proceed to the exercises of this sequence.

The exercises have been given names that describe the movements. The reader will find that this will enable him to fix the exercise quickly and lastingly in mind.

THE TOE JUMP 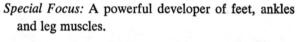 *Special Focus:* A powerful developer of feet, ankles and leg muscles.

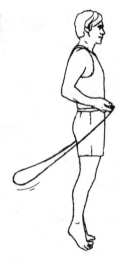

Position: From regular jump-rope stance, raise yourself to a high tiptoe position, with your body weight forward and entirely upon the under-toes.

Action: Perform regular jump/turns while on high tiptoe.

THE HEEL
JUMP

Special Focus: A developer for torso shock-absorber action.

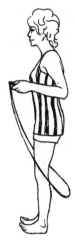

Position: From regular jump-rope stance, lift forward part of foot off floor. Place weight entirely upon heel pad.

Action: Perform regular jump/turns while remaining far back on the heel pad.

THE ELEVATOR

Special Focus: Hip-girdle, pelvic-area and small-of-back conditioner.

Position: Basic jump-rope stance.

Action: Dip gradually down, bending from the knees, while performing regular jump/turns. Sink to deep crouch. Rise gradually while continuing jump/turns.

THE
KANGAROO

Special Focus: More intense hip-girdle, pelvic-area conditioner.

Position: Semicrouch, with knees forward, buttocks out.

Action: Dip down to complete crouch and leap forward during the performance of regular jump/turns.

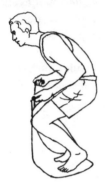 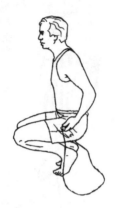

THE WIDE WING

Special Focus: High-level torso conditioner.

Position: From regular jump/turn stance, raise arms 45 degrees upward and outward to the sides.

Action: Perform rope turns from this position and jump high to clear shortened rope span.

THE MOUSE

(Performed with THE GAZELLE)
Special Focus: Reflex developer from low to sudden high level of bodily exertion.

Position: Basic jump-rope stance.

Action: A series of small quick steps (4) forward during jump/turns and these steps extending into . . .

THE GAZELLE   *Special Focus:* Thigh, pelvis and buttock conditioner.

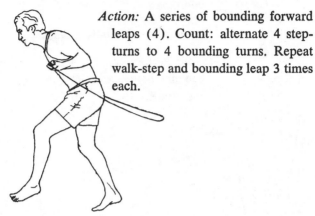

Action: A series of bounding forward leaps (4). Count: alternate 4 step-turns to 4 bounding turns. Repeat walk-step and bounding leap 3 times each.

THE SPACE MAN   *Special Focus:* Strengthener of large thigh and buttock muscles; conditions pelvis.

Position: Basic jump-rope stance.

Action: Sink to lowest knee-bent level and launch into high bounding leap during regular jump/turns.

THE DOUBLE SPIN-JUMP   *Special Focus:* Improved high-level muscular co-ordination.

Position: Basic jump stance.

Action: Double hand-spin for each single high jump.

THE CRISS-
CROSS

Special Focus: Improved timing and high-level coordination.

Position: Basic jump/turn stance.

Action: Perform regular jump/turns while crossing and uncrossing arms at chest level to criss-cross rope spins.

THE
MARATHON

Special Focus: Endurance.

Position: Basic jump stance. Hand-spin. One-step.

Action: Smooth, relaxed motions; consistent *medium* tempo.

MASTERING
THE INTER-
MEDIATE
JUMP-ROPE
EXERCISES

Once again it is urged that you do not leap too hastily into the prescribed weekly schedules. The same procedure that accompanies the mastery of the standard exercises is recommended.

- Learn the new exercise movements.
- Smooth out their execution so they can be performed without interruption.
- Allow for gradual body adjustment to more demanding exercises.

The orientation session to achieve this will consist of:

- Four jump-rope exercises per session.
- Except for THE MARATHON, all exercises will be divided into 4 sets with a jump count of 10 for each. This will permit a rest between each set.
- The exercise of each session will be considered mastered when the 4 sets of jump/turns are completed with no more than 2 misses. When a miss occurs, the set in which the miss is made is begun again.
- Repeat the same orientation exercise session until all of its exercises are mastered.
- Rest means full breathing recovery throughout the orientation period.

Do NOT continue any orientation exercise session beyond a period of 10 minutes of actual jumping time, exclusive of rest.

Do NOT exercise for more than 3 complete sessions in any one day during the orientation period.

Do NOT move into the next exercise until the preceding ones have been mastered.

THE
FUNMAKER
APPROACH

If you find yourself stymied during any single exercise session, if you are too impatient to perfect any exercise, or if you are missing too often and having to start again, I recommend the *Funmaker* approach.

1. Stop all attempts to complete the session according to the rules.

2. Take up the rope and just jump for the *fun* of it. Do THE TRAIN and THE MARATHON if you like, or neither one. Play with the movements—the two-step and one-step; the arm-spin and hand-spin; the ball-of-foot step, toe-jump step, flat-foot step. Do any jump-rope maneuver that comes to mind or one you do well. Fill in the number of times you need to conclude the session.

3. Go to Part III, *Funmaker Fitness,* and have a ball.

4. Take up the regular session next time. And if it doesn't work out, go back to the *Funmaker* section. In time, it will work out. Do not stubbornly insist upon perfection too soon. Forcing the issue will only throw you out of rhythm and add to the difficulty. With the *Funmaker* approach, you are jumping and earning the benefit of circulatory exercise. And . . . you are improving your technique.

ORIENTA-
TION
SESSIONS

Two of the four exercises in each session (after the first) will be repeats. The exerciser is therefore once more expected to master two new positions within each session. Again, THE TRAIN and THE MARATHON are the repeats—the first, as a warm-up and to refine jump/turn skills and rhythms; the second, an incentive exercise, which will serve as an improvement measure. It is the only one of the four exercises with a varying count.

Unless otherwise noted, the exercises are to be performed in the *Two-step, Arm-spin, Ball-of-foot position,* at *Medium tempo.*

First Session	THE TRAIN	THE TOE JUMP	THE HEEL JUMP	THE MARATHON
	10 slow 2/s	Count 10 Rest	Count 10 Rest	Count 200+
	20 medium 2/s	Count 10 Rest	Count 10 Rest	Maximum Count: 350
	10 fast 1/s	Count 10 Rest	Count 10 Rest	
		Count 10 Rest	Count 10 Rest	

Second Session	THE TRAIN	THE ELEVATOR	THE KANGAROO	THE MARATHON
	10 slow 2/s	Count 10 Rest	Count 10 Rest	Count 200+
	20 medium 2/s	Count 10 Rest	Count 10 Rest	Maximum Count: 350
	10 fast 1/s	Count 10 Rest	Count 10 Rest	
		Count 10 Rest	Count 10 Rest	

Third Session	THE TRAIN	THE MOUSE	THE GAZELLE	THE MARATHON
	10 slow 2/s	Count 10 Rest	Count 10 Rest	Count 200+
	20 medium 2/s	Count 10 Rest	Count 10 Rest	Maximum Count: 350
	10 fast 1/s	Count 10 Rest	Count 10 Rest	
		Count 10 Rest	Count 10 Rest	

Fourth Session	THE TRAIN	THE WIDE WING	THE SPACE MAN	THE MARATHON
	10 slow 2/s	Count 10 Rest	Count 10 Rest	Count 200+
	20 medium 2/s	Count 10 Rest	Count 10 Rest	Maximum Count: 350
	10 fast 1/s	Count 10 Rest	Count 10 Rest	
		Count 10 Rest	Count 10 Rest	

Fifth Session	THE TRAIN	THE CRISS-CROSS	THE DOUBLE-SPIN	THE MARATHON
	10 slow 2/s	Count 10 Rest	Count 10 Rest	Count 200+
	20 medium 2/s	Count 10 Rest	Count 10 Rest	Maximum Count: 350
	10 fast 1/s	Count 10 Rest	Count 10 Rest	
		Count 10 Rest	Count 10 Rest	

REGULAR
WEEKLY
SCHEDULES

- *Minimum* number of jump-rope workouts: 6 per week, once daily. One rest day.
    Recommended: 12 per week, twice daily.
- Exercise Schedules A and B, which follow, are to be performed on alternate days.
- Unless otherwise noted, all exercises are to be performed at *medium tempo, ball-of-foot position, arm-spin position, two-step.*
- Continue with intermediate jump-rope ex-

ercise schedule a *minimum* of 8 successive weeks. Those satisfied with this level of activity may permanently maintain it. Others may proceed to the advanced level.

INTERMEDIATE EXERCISE SCHEDULE A

Energy Output Approximately 160+ Calories
This is a 15 minute exercise session.* But there is no need for clock-watching. All you need to do is follow the count given with each exercise.

Warm-up   THE TRAIN

Count 20 slow (two-step)
Count 30 medium (two-step)
Count 20 fast (one-step)
    Rest

Set 1 THE TOE JUMP	*Set 2* THE HEEL JUMP
Count 30	Count 30
Rest	Rest
Count 30	Count 30
Rest	Rest

Set 3 THE ELEVATOR	*Set 4* THE KANGAROO
Count 30	Count 30
Rest	Rest
Count 30	Count 30
Rest	Rest

* With each exercise, unless otherwise noted, a count of 30 (two-step) equals approximately 23 seconds. Rest is an equal interval. Each exercise performed twice for a total time per set of 1½ minutes + *The Train* + *The Marathon* equals complete total of 15 minutes (approximately).

Set 5	THE MOUSE	Set 6	THE GAZELLE
	Count 30		Count 30
	Rest		Rest
	Count 30		Count 30
	Rest		Rest

Set 7	THE WIDE WING	Set 8	THE SPACE MAN
	Count 30		Count 30
	Rest		Rest
	Count 30		Count 30
	Rest		Rest

Endurance Jump THE MARATHON
Continuous one-step.
Keep a record of each session.
Attempt to exceed it each time to eventually peak at a count of 500.

INTERMEDIATE EXERCISE SCHEDULE B
Energy Output
    Approximately 175+ Calories
Same instructions as in Schedule A apply.

Warm-up THE TRAIN
Count 20 slow (two-step)
Count 30 medium (two-step)
Count 20 fast (two-step)

Set 1	THE TOE JUMP	Set 2	THE HEEL JUMP
	Count 30		Count 30
	Rest		Rest
	Count 30		Count 30
	Rest		Rest

Set 3	THE ELEVATOR	*Set 4*	THE KANGAROO
	Count 30		Count 30
	Rest		Rest
	Count 30		Count 30
	Rest		Rest
Set 5	THE CRISS-CROSS	*Set 6*	THE DOUBLE-SPIN
	Count 30		Count 30
	Rest		Rest
	Count 30		Count 30
	Rest		Rest

Endurance Jump   THE MARATHON
Continuous one-step.
Keep a record of each session.
Attempt to exceed it each time to eventually peak at a count of 500.

CHAPTER 11   AdvANCEd jump-ROpE
EXERCiSE SchEdulES

You ARE READY to take the big step into the advanced jump-rope exercises if you have:

- Kept up weekly workouts with the intermediate exercise schedules for *no less than* 8 weeks.
- Found progressive signs of physical improvement and are desirous of still-more demanding activity.
- Been able to come to the 500 MARATHON count.
- Been given the go-ahead on the basis of your Pulse Test (see p. 68) results.

This time, you have no new exercises to master! It becomes a matter of refined proficiency, more precise coordination and more challenging programing of the same movements. Interestingly, after a few weeks of workouts at this level, you will find that you are *putting out the least effort and performing at the highest level.* It is the signal that your body has once again made an adjustment on a higher plateau of physical development. The new balance and deeper rhythms have settled down to become your norm. A further reward for this attainment: *it will require about the same time to perform the advanced schedules and maintain superior fitness levels as it did the intermediate schedules!*

Since you are familiar with the exercise movements and are physically fit, the customary exercise orientation period has been eliminated.

ADVANCED EXERCISE SCHEDULE A

Energy Output Approximately 200+ Calories
This is a 15+ minute exercise session.* But there is no need for clock-watching. All you need to do is to follow the count given with each exercise.

Warm-up THE TRAIN

Count 20 slow (two-step)
Count 40 medium (one-step)
Count 60 fast (running-step)
  Rest

* With each exercise, unless otherwise noted, a count of 40 (two-step) equals approximately ½ minute. Rest at this stage of physical fitness is about *half* this interval. Each exercise performed twice for a total time 1½ minutes + *The Train* (1½ minutes) + *The Marathon* (average 600 count one-step) equals approximately 5 minutes.

Set 1	THE SAG	*Set 2*	THE PEACOCK
	Count 40		Count 40
	Rest		Rest
	Count 40		Count 40
	Rest		Rest

		Set 4	THE CRISS-CROSS
Set 3	THE GROUCHO		
	Count 40		Count 40
	Rest		Rest
	Count 40		Count 40
	Rest		Rest

Set 5	THE DOUBLE-SPIN	*Set 6*	THE PRANCE
	Count 40		Count 40
	Rest		Rest
	Count 40		Count 40
	Rest		Rest

Endurance Jump THE MARATHON

Continuous. Jumper permitted to change jump steps and vary rate over 500+ count.

(Two-, one-, running-steps for coasting, resting, accelerating.) Keep a record of each session. Try to exceed it.

ADVANCED EXERCISE SCHEDULE B

This is the peak activity level of *The Jump-Rope Exercise System*. Those attaining this level may participate in the more rigorous types of endurance activities.

- The exercises are the same.
- The counts are the same (except for THE MARATHON).

- The difference lies in combining the exercise sets. It is possible, depending upon the condition and endurance of the exerciser, to go through all sets with one rest, or none.
- THE TRAIN and THE MARATHON are still to be performed as separate exercises with appropriate rests.

Warm-up   THE TRAIN
(as on page 41)

Set 1   THE SAG

Count 80
No break
in between

Set 2   THE PEACOCK

Count 80
No break
in between

Set 4   THE CRISS-CROSS

Count 80
No break
in between

Set 3   THE GROUCHO

Count 80
No break
in between
Rest to
recover as
necessary

Set 5   THE DOUBLE-SPIN

Count 80
No break
in between

Set 6   THE PRANCE

Count 80
No break
in between
Rest to
recover as
necessary

Endurance Jump   THE MARATHON
(as on page 41)

jump-rope exercise
pulse test

WITH REGULAR performance of *The Jump-Rope Exercise System,* the benefits will become readily observable. Comments will be made about your improved appearance and more energetic approach to living. But because the System is designed to have deep-down internal benefits, it is convenient to have a device that you can use to gauge your progress and its effect upon your circulatory system. The Pulse Test, a simple and an accurate one, adequately fulfills this function.

- Begin using the Pulse Test when you start with the weekly standard exercise schedule.
- Repeat the Pulse Test after every three weeks of regular exercise sessions.
- The pulse should be taken each time following the same exercise. THE MARATHON is recommended as a test exercise.

PULSE
TEST
PROCEDURE

1. Do not take any exercise for at least 15 minutes preceding the test.

2. Follow the given MARATHON exercise count* according to your level of progress:

	Standard	Intermediate	Advanced
1st Week	Count: 50	Count: 200	Count: 500
4th Week	Count: 100	Count: 300	Count: 700
7th-8th Week	Count: 200	Count: 500	Count: 1000

3. Be seated for 2 minutes.

4. Count out the pulse for ½ minute. Double this for the 1-minute rate.

What to Look For: a steady *decrease* in the pulse rate. This will show that less effort is required by your system to perform the same or increased activity. It is an indication that the internal organs are coordinating better and putting out with a higher efficiency. Presently, as the conditioning of your body improves, the pulse rate will level off at the newer, more effective rate.

Remember: your pulse count is another mark of your individuality. There are differences from person to person. Comparing your pulse rate with someone else's can be instructive only for a physician. For the purposes of this test, comparisons are significant only if they are made on the basis of your own pulse rate.

---

* The raised count is to be used even if you have reached this count in your regular exercise sessions. If not, repeat the same test level until you do.

PART III **funmaker fitness**

CHAPTER 13 **jump for fun and fitness**

I MUST apologize for starting off the Funmaker section on a serious note. But my intentions are *honorable,* as will soon become evident, in this attempt to encourage you to "let your hair down" as you take up your jump rope.

In pursuing a very hectic, progress-oriented lifestyle, most of us rather stubbornly cling to the attitude that nothing can really be good for us unless it is quite serious and involves a bit of ordeal. "Business [which, significantly, is derived from busy-ness] before pleasure" is an integral part of the industrious heritage that has given us our incredibly *industrialized* environment. In the words of that popular TV commercial, we have come "a long way, baby." But our bodies would never have made it without those occasional breaks for fun, for enjoyment, which are re-creative and recreational. The more deeply invigorating and joyous the release, the healthier the tempo pickup of the vital body rhythms.

Fun is an exercise of *feeling action,* our deepest and most natural body rhythms, in contrast to that process uniquely human—*thinking action.* Thinking is our way of overriding the feeling signals and often repressing them entirely. True, it has given us an exceedingly advanced civilization, but it has also separated us from the rhythms of nature and our *natural* body rhythms.

These brief excerpts from Rockefeller University scientist René Dubos' studies on the subject are very much to the point:

> Most functions of the human body exhibit marked daily rhythms affecting such things as the composition of the blood and the urine, the secretion of hormones, deep body temperature and blood flow. . . . Technology can mask some of the environmental forces under which human evolution took place, but it does not thereby abolish the biological rhythms that were woven into the human fabric during evolution. This dissociation between the two kinds of rhythms is a very recent experience for the human race. . . .[6]

The point is clear enough and unarguable, with so much evidence in our everyday lives to substantiate it. It is a major problem all our lives, on every level, and I certainly am not about to offer up the jump rope as a crusade to save the world. But we *can* make a small start, which is not small for *you,* toward the revitalization of your body rhythms. Let's face it: the human body was simply not made for so complex an environment. For

[6] René Dubos, "The Human Environment," *Science Journal,* vol. 5A, no. 4 (October 1969), p. 76.

example—and sometimes cold statistics can have a sobering effect—in our highly automated and electronic times, the human nervous system is assaulted by some 10,000 sensory impressions every single second! The tempo is set by our machines, and our underexercised bodies are left to react mentally. No wonder there is so much anxiety and draining nervous tension. And no wonder that the author of the classic *On Aggression,* Dr. Konrad Lorenz, looks toward human laughter to save the world.

So for heaven's and your health's sake, have some fun with the jump rope *and* this Funmaker section. Adolescence is not a bad word or a bad stage from which to recapture some *joie de vivre,* so that you need not irascibly protest, as George Bernard Shaw did, the waste of youth on the young.

AT HOME   *For Housewives:* medical science has informed us that tiredness comes in two varieties. One is the kind that comes from a great deal of continuous, very heavy labor. Sleep is the remedy. The other is a common household variety. It comes from such things as performing the same, hardly varying daily routine: doing a great many boring, small chores; a limited demand upon the mental powers; the use of the same sets of muscles in doing daily tasks— the lack of surprise or of the unexpected, and a low level of emotional stimulation. These bring on the condition of *psychological fatigue.* And you know the symptoms: drowsiness; lack of energy; desire to sit and rest; the watching of TV for long hours; or oversleep. The *prescription:* the deep-down rhythmical circulatory *jump-rope exercise.*

The way to go at it is to do a quick review of your daily routine. For instance, it's time to do the laundry. When you go to the basement or wherever you have your washing machine, take your jump rope with you. Try THE STIFF (See p. 40) or:

THE RUN
AND RINSE
A cycle of running steps followed by a cycle of one-steps. A jump count of 10 for each. Rest and repeat 3 times.

If "no thanks" is your reaction to these exercises, go ahead on your own and do THE FREE FLY, which is a relaxed, anything-goes/anyway-you-do-it jump style. And if you think THE TALK-A-THON TWIRL might be more congenial in tandem, invite a friend or friends over to jump in for a twirl, one-at-a-time. If you have one of those tight little apartments and use the local laundromat, it might surprise you to discover a friend or two who will be really taken with the jump-rope idea and get into the act.

THE
TALK-A-THON
TWIRL
A nice casual beginning with a gentle, unlaboring two-step, which allows you to still react and respond to choice bits of gossip. A handy warm-up that doesn't put a silencer on you. Jump to count 10 and rest, three sets. Jump to count 20 and rest, three sets.

THIRTY
DAYS HATH
SEPTEMBER
Rhythmically recite and jump each month, as far as you can go without missing. It won't take you more than a week or two before you can do a complete year—in 5 minutes. Talk about jet-propelled!

Then there's mealtime preparation. The ingredients are mixed and on the stove or in the oven, and here's your opportunity to take up your jump rope. Now's a good time to crouch and do THE GROUCHO (p. 36). Nobody's looking. Follow with THE CHAPLIN (p. 39), toes pointed out. Both are ridiculous but absolutely fabulous exercises—and guaranteed laughmakers in any group participation.

If these movements are not your cup of tea, do THE FREE FLY, with our compliments. To keep it rhythmical, why don't you tap out, "Now is the time for all good men to come to the aid of their party," as your jump refrain.

How about that time in the day when the morning "rush hour" is over? The man of the house has left for the job and the kids have gone to school. You're still not more than 37 percent awake. Even the second cup of coffee doesn't seem to quite do the trick. Try the jump rope and see what happens. Start out just the way you feel. Do THE SAG (p. 34); next try THE PEACOCK (p. 37).

Where moments ago you felt sapped, ready to tumble back into bed, you will be astonished by your wide-eyed awakening. A splash of water on your face, a comb through your hair, a dab of makeup and—the day doesn't look too bad after all.

The Friendly Enemies of Fitness: these enemies are all around you, within your reach. Everyone is familiar with their *friendly* side—wonderful comfort and convenience. But few of us are aware of the damaging effects of having too much of a good thing. Let's consider the more prominent of these friendly enemies of fitness.

The family car. What a boon for getting about. You sit yourself down and a toe on the gas pedal does the rest. Remember walking? Alas, it's rapidly becoming a relic of bygone times. Your jump rope should be remembered and brought into play after the car trip around the corner to mail a letter.

The sofa. The temptation to lie down and stretch out when fatigue is of the psychological variety can just lead to more and more tiredness. Another reason for your jump rope.

The refrigerator. How easily the door swings open to an absolute wonderworld of abundance for mealtimes. But in between times, it also swings. Why not just drape the jump rope over the top of the refrigerator as a reminder and "skip" this friendly enemy?

The television set. Let us direct our attention to perhaps the most insidious friendly enemy of them all—the mesmerizing eye that exerts its ultimate influence in the evening when all submit and lie quiescent beneath its bright and sometimes baleful glare.

But here is a way to have your "TV cake" and eat it too! If you adopt this jump-rope routine, you may languish on the sofa and watch to your heart's content. You will sleep restfully and awaken refreshed and fit each morning after. There is no need to intrude upon your favorite programs with—The TV TURNABOUT. The jump rope is to be taken up only at the following times: during commercials, station breaks, dull spots in the talk shows, the weather report.

I am not suggesting that *all* of these moments be used for ropejumping. The rope should be reached for at intervals when the mood so inclines. Or when tedium and drowsiness show signs of bringing on too-early sleep. If one were to make a jump session of only the weather report and a commercial or two or intervals in a talk show, it would fill the daily exercise quota. With an exercise as vigorous as ropejumping, the 7-minute minimum can work wonders. Because jump-rope activity is an amusement, the exercise-minutes literally fly by.

And since several members of the family are likely to be present during The TV Turn-about, the fun can be contagious. Here are several playtime feats and contests to get everybody into the act: The Exceeder (p. 105), The Jet Spin (p. 105), The Slow-Down (p. 104) and The Kangaroo (p. 53).

The Free Fly may be substituted for any of these exercises—or perhaps a tandem jump with a partner, and feats, such as The Double-Spin (p. 55). Reading through the other sections will soon equip the jumper with a repertoire of his own favorites.

WHILE BACK AT THE OFFICE

For executives, secretaries, advertising brainstormers, and effete intellectual snobs. So many books by authorities on the subject make reference to the human body as "a perfect machine." The powerful muscles designed to perform heavy work and absorb the necessary oxygen to turn the body's fuel into energy keep the life-giving cycle of all the internal organs in rhythmic balance. The body is, we are given to understand, ideally designed for man's natural environment.

How, then, to explain the current, all-pervasive state of physical *un*fitness? The fault is to be found in the phrase "natural environment." Apparently, the body *is* a perfect machine, but for a time and place that no longer exist. We have wheels to replace legs, machines to replace arms and muscle power, thermostatically controlled buildings that make the body's own temperature controls obsolete. Daylight comes along, and the human body is geared for the physical activity it needs to remain sound and healthy. But by the millions, we enter the city, take an elevator up to an office *to sit down* and go to work. It really isn't an absolute essential to get up from the chair, even to be fed. The telephone produces a convenient lunch delivery. So what happens to the work of the muscles, the intake of the oxygen, the blood circulation in this wonderful machine?

Practically everyone is aware of the problem —and also the way to overcome it: exercise. But few seem to have the time or the inclination. This is natural because the *capacity* drops as the level of *performance* drops. Physical activity that might once have been simple gets to be a real ordeal. There is that long day at the office, during which time most of the damage is being done. Any intention of making up for it later in the evening with exercise fades with the passing hours.

A way out of the dilemma is to get your exercise in the office!

Did you know that there are generally two letdown periods in the day for most office workers? One in the morning, about 11:00, and the other toward the late afternoon, about 3:30. Not surprising, now that we know something about psychological fatigue. The jump rope can be used for a lift out of these doldrums.

There is a special Office Jump Week Schedule on page 137 of *The Jump-Rope Personalizer,* if you want to organize your office jump-rope routines. Then again, you may prefer to play it by ear and jump as the mood and occasion command. You're the jumpmaster!

THE HEAD   A great eye-opener. Assume a basic jump position
SWIVEL   and swivel the head loosely and continuously while jumping. This will loosen the muscles of the neck, and the jump action will stimulate the blood flow to the face and the brain. Jump to count 20. Rest and repeat once or twice more as needed.

THE HEAD SWIVEL is a great aid before a big company meeting, a confrontation with the boss or any situation calling for maximum alertness. For the typewriter-befogged secretary with a male lunchdate, it is truly a secret weapon. Several determined jumps and she is as ebullient as the champagne cocktail she will surely receive as a tribute.

And after doing her own "daily dozens," if she wishes to do her boss a good turn, she could leave him her rope with a note describing the following exercises for the stiff back and "sleepy legs" of the close-to-retirement executive: THE TRAIN, THE GREYHOUND and THE SWAYBACK (see pp. 37, 38 and 41 respectively).

For the more youthful and ambitious male

executive, to THE PEACOCK, THE GREYHOUND and THE SWAYBACK may be added THE PRANCE (p. 36) and THE SPACE MAN (p. 55).

The choices are many, with a more or less organized routine, as the exerciser prefers. For those interested in a rounded program, a selection of any three *standards,* beginning with THE TRAIN and ending with THE MARATHON, is recommended. A jumping interval of 5 minutes is sufficient. If such exercisers wish to design a program with a more specific concentration on the back, thighs, abdomen or other special weak spots, the section on *The Jump-Rope Personalizer* should be referred to. For THE FREE FLY, anything goes. They may prefer, instead, to participate in some of the jump games described along the way.

For working girls, secretaries, receptionists, switchboard operators and others of their beleaguered clan, that sit-down look can be particularly devastating. Several jump-rope revivers: THE STAR-SWALLOW (p. 38), THE KANGAROO (p. 53), and:

THE BAREFOOT BOUNCE   One of the quickest ways to liven up and restore the bounce is to kick off the shoes and, with the jump rope, perform as follows—THE FREE FLY and count to 20, swinging into the one-legged jump, alternating right and left for another 20. The toes will tingle, the calves and thighs firm up and the upper torso shake to new trimness.

If you're a joiner, your turn is coming up. The game and participation type of jumping does require work-break periods like morning coffee, post-lunch gabfest, afternoon coffee, and so on. For such times, you might wish to bring in a double length of clothesline. Remember the sidewalk jump routine when two turners would stand at opposite ends and spin for the center jumper or jumpers?

THE
SECRETARY-
POOL JUMP
Use either a single rope or two ropes, spun simultaneously clockwise and counterclockwise. Invite one or two adventurous jumpers at a time, ready to give it a whirl.

Ideal for office participation are these familiars: THE EXCEEDER, THE JET SPIN, THE SLOW-DOWN (See pp. 104 and 105). An office competition, which is certain to continue with heightening excitement, is to be found under the section, *Competitive Jump-Rope Events.* Start in immediately to shoot for your proficiency level—*Fleebee, Cloudbuster, Jumpronaut*—or for the ultimate, *Space Swami.*

You can play . . .

FOLLOW
THE JUMP-
LEADER
Indoor version, with the jumpers remaining stationary and imitating the jump movement changes of the leader. By scanning the various chapters, the jump-leader can build up a repertoire tough enough to frustrate any group of followers.

JUMPMAN'S
BLUFF
A simple, fun game. A small chalk circle is drawn around the jumper's feet, and he or she is blind-

folded. The object is to jump as long as possible without crossing the line. Large linoleum squares can be used instead of the chalk circle.

Skill jumps such as FLIP THE CAP, from the section on *Jump-Rope Games and Contests,* can be used with coffee-time treats or lunchtime cocktails for the prizes. See other gamblers' jump games in the same section. Jump games for office parties are also described there.

THE
JUMP-ROPE
TRAVELER
Future or Culture Shock, those popular phrases of author Alvin Toffler, have everything to do with the too-quick pace of change to which our bodies cannot adjust promptly enough. Whether it happens in familiar places of work and living because of the electronic tempo of events or because of jetting into new surroundings and altered daily rituals, the effects are similar: the disordering of the vital body rhythms.

So why not *do* something about it by getting down to where nature is at? Take a jump rope along and put it to use in *harmonizing* the body rhythms. Handily tucked into a suitcase, a shoulder bag, a business portfolio or even a roomy purse, a jump rope can be conveniently retrieved for those relaxing jump interludes.

You needn't be thinking of the synchronizing effect on heartbeat, circulation, oxygen intake, muscle frame and vital organ stimulation. Jump for sheer joy, and let all of the rest come over you like a tranquilizing wave.

Try THE RAILROAD RUMBLE, a jump to the

rhythm of the rails. You hardly need more than standing-room-only, and it's a sure way to attract a kindred soul or two. Between or during brief rest stops, spin out the lingering rhythms. At bus stops on Greyhound trips, a minute or two of vigorous jump/turns can quickly buoy up body and spirits and put an end to hobbling legs, brain drain and creaking back.

For those destination blues and blahs, break out the jump rope. Relax. Let your head droop, shoulders sag and legs go rubbery. Pick up a simple tune in your head, pleasant and easygoing and take up the jump tempo. *Boomp-boomp-a-doomp, boomp-boomp-a-doomp . . . Boomp.* No thoughts, no special goals or objectives. Up and down, that's what it's all about. And be wise enough to go along with it. Visualize your head as a big, overexpanded balloon, and let the pressure ease out of it until that tight band around your temples is gone.

Now, if it's time for sleep, slide right into THE NIGHTCAP jump-rope exercise. But if activity, business or social, is on your agenda, gradually step up the rhythm to the level of a fast spin-out and then ease down the tempo again. Keep up these short sequences, slow to a fast, wide-eyed tempo, igniting deep-down energy sparks. I call this THE No-Doz. When it starts to work for you, hit the shower, brisk and needlepoint, and come to refreshed and exuberant life. Use the towel as if you mean it. Don't spare the cologne. And from here, you're on your own with your best foot forward.

THE NIGHTCAP   Beginning with THE RAILROAD RUMBLE, do not go into the stepped-up No-Doz, but continue with that same soporific spin. A regular, unchanging, slow-to-moderate tempo, occasionally letting your eyelids droop, with tension sneaking out from behind your eyeballs. If your breathing becomes labored, rest by leaning back against the wall or bedstead, with your eyes closed. Once your breathing becomes regular again, repeat the sequence.

It works like magic and is ideal for the inveterate or occasional insomniac. The limbs grow heavier, a nightshade slipping hypnotically over the brain, until all you want to do is flop into bed. But tease yourself a while with THE NIGHTCAP treatment until hitting the sack seems like the world's sweetest prospect.

THE TURNPIKE TWIRL A jump-rope intermission that is the innovation of Murray R., a salesman constantly on the move and one of the world's greatest proselytizers of this fitness activity. His favorite line in persuading others to try ropejumping is one I long ago plagiarized: "It is the one exercise you will swear *by* instead of *at!*"

His routine calls for two hours of driving, interrupted by jump-rope stops, "much to the amusement of everybody looking on," Murray avows, "but with more jump-rope disciples left behind me than you can shake a billboard at!" Once seriously afflicted with what he calls an occupational hazard of those inactivated behind the wheel of a car for long, uninterrupted hours of driving—chronic leg cramps—Murray attributes to this jump-rope routine his "legs like a dancer's and more energy and drive than a Mack truck!"

- If possible, stop where there is some green-ery that maintains a good oxygen supply in the air.
- Breathe deeply—all the way in, all the way out—20 times.
- The Ropeless Jump-Offs: THE KNEE JUMP, THE APACHE JUMP, THE FLING-WING—15 times each (*See* pp. 24, 25 and 26 respec-tively.)
- THE SAG, THE KANGAROO, THE TOE JUMP—30 times each. (*See* pp. ?§ 52 and 53 re-spectively.)
- THE MARATHON. (*See* p. 41.)

"It is a fitness formula that will get you where you are going in better shape than when you left," is Murray's guarantee. And it is one which I en-thusiastically endorse.

THE
JUMP-ROPE
FANTASY
TRAVELER

This is for those people who are happier when they aim at an ambitious goal. It keeps them more in-terested in their day-to-day performance. This is where the idea for *The Jump-Rope Fantasy Traveler* comes in.

Pick your favorite European country. England? France? A Scandinavian country? Tack up a map with a mileage scale of it on the wall of your pre-ferred "jump room." Now, let's estimate that the energy for each jump covers the equivalent of a 3-foot pace. That would give us about 1820 paces or *jumps* to the mile. Let's be sporting and use 1500 paces for a round figure.

How far will you travel in a month? Three months? Six months? Jumping across to Sicily. It would make quite an item for conversation, or if you are more patriotic, how about across the state of Virginia? Or would you say that the whole idea smacks of madness?

DOWN AT THE COMMUNE

(For creative think-tankers, artists, revolutionaries and commune folk.) THE COMMUNE JUMP-IN: try it at sunrise, sunset or around an evening outdoor fire. If you want group rapport that you haven't had before, this is the prescription from one of my former jump-rope fitness enthusiasts, S.M., a charming "dropout" New York City social worker and presently a member of a California commune. This group jump-in is borrowed from her correspondence describing it to me. It was her own idea and she writes of sunrise and sunset as the more inspirational times of day when she has conducted her jump-ins. I suggest night, around an outdoor fire, as well. And the routine calls for no talking, no *vocal* expression at all.

It begins with a jump rope being passed silently from hand to hand, until one member of the group feels the urge and then begins to jump, using his own style and tempo. After an interval it is passed along to another member of the group, until all members have had an opportunity to jump. Then another rope is passed around and *two* members of the group jump in relation to each other until their rhythms are in unison. The jumping couples, one and then another, face each other and, writes S.M., "it soon becomes a ritualistic communion of body rhythms, a kind of inner orchestration, each playing out his vibrations to the other."

But to sum up her lengthy account, the ritual becomes communal with *everybody* jumping. And

S.M.'s claim is that it builds up to a "communal group sensitivity, a sort of subconscious wavelength on which an extraordinary sense of closeness is possible." How effective this is, I cannot say. But the group fun, the fitness benefits and the stimulation of the deep bio-rhythms should be fully rewarding on their own account.

THE JUMP-ROPE REVOLUTION This is the kind of *revolution* that refers to the number of jump/turns per minute. But in these days of on- and off-campus demonstrations for community affairs, women's (or anyone else's) lib and so on, a potent symbol for peace, for cooling edgy "vibes," can be—*The Rope of Hope*. Taking the lead from S.M.'s jump-in and the effect upon group body rhythms, I suggest that some jump ropes be passed around. Then watch it happen almost magically: people joyously jumping and lots of easy laughter as the body rhythms fall into synchronism. Maybe some of our more ebullient politicians will be trying it next as they hit the stump with the corniest campaign slogan of all time—"Those who jump together, stump together." Or vice versa.

The one thread of sanity in this inanity is the principle of bringing group body rhythms into harmonious accord. It is the underlying meaning of that vague expression that the "vibes are right. . . ."

THE ZEN ORBIT This is the jump-rope exercise devised as a "sure-fire mental refresher" by Greg R., a computer-company executive assigned to creative development. Combining the jump-rope activity with his interest in Zen Buddhism, this exercise has proved marvelously effective as a creative re-energizer for several others I have passed it along to, including a novelist in his sixties, a rock musician and songwriter of reputation and a young woman partner of a New York advertising firm.

A part of the practice of Zen meditation is to concentrate on an idea that transcends the logical, such as the instruction, "Imagine the sound of one hand clapping." Such a practice, it is said, helps to clear the mind and open the way to inspiring insights. Greg found that when he was mentally blocked on a problem, the continuous rhythmic cadence of the jump rope applied in a specific way could enhance the Zen meditation effect. This is his procedure:

- Close your eyes but not so tightly that there is a feeling of eye stress.
- Feel your pulse beat and use it as your jump-rope tempo. You will soon be aware of your heartbeat and let it be your metronome.
- Presently, the effect is one of being "totally enveloped in your own body presence, as if it were a vast ocean with the pulses as flowing tides."
- It is when the dividing line of inside-and-out of the body and the universe around it begins to fade that the desired response is being achieved. And the sensation is that of all thought and idea emerging from somewhere in the center of the body.
- When this is felt, the jumper is to lie down, preferably, or slump into a tilt-back desk chair and maintain this state as if in a semi-trance.

"When you get to be especially good at it," Greg states, "all kinds of fresh images, ideas, thoughts, begin to push their way up into the conscious mind."

But at the very least, as others I have taught this jump-rope exercise to have testified, it does help clear the head of prior thoughts and ideas that could not be shaken loose.

UP A DOWN STAIRCASE

This is another jump-rope improvisation of Greg R.'s, one he also refers to as THE FRUSTRATION WALTZ. He recommends it "to work off those built-up aggressions when confronted with a moment of unreason by the boss or some business colleague." And I agree on general principle that when frustration takes over for any reason and you feel like you are fit to be tied, a jump/turn diversion is a great way to untie yourself by releasing the pent-up energy.

Greg's images—this one, of jumping as if continuously descending an upward moving escalator—have more method than madness. The idea is to divert the mind from thoughts that continue to build up frustration at the same time that vigorous physical activity is helping to return harmonious body rhythms.

As for the jump-rope exercise, it is similar to THE ZEN ORBIT, but with the image changed. It is therefore equally effective as a creative mental stimulator.

I attribute the very conspicuous mood-changing influence of jump-rope activity to its alteration of the body rhythms. It should not be surprising, really, since these rhythms are directly related to our body chemistry and our brain-wave patterns. And because of this, we would all be a lot better off reaching for the jump rope rather than casually resorting to the arsenal of mood-changing drugs—"uppies, downies" or what have you.

We know not only from various tribal dances that rhythmic body movements are used to influence emotions, but also from certain religious practices, such as those of the "whirling dervishes." These holy men rhythmically whirl their bodies about until they achieve trancelike states reportedly similar to drug highs.

So how about recommending for someone feeling *low,* the jump-rope high?

CHAPTER 14 **jump-rope games and contests**

IF YOU ARE a gamester, playboy or competitive-event type, you are the most anti-exercise of all. You'd rather do anything *but*. Even those who go in for the competitive events, strenuous as they may be, do it for the excitement. The exercise is a bonus. You'll want to bring yourself up to the intermediate jump-rope level of fitness and proficiency for these games.

GAMES AND FEATS JUMP-ROPE TAG: The person designated "it" runs after other participants. Everyone engaged in the game must be jumping rope continuously. The tag is considered effective only if the rope of the it man snaps another's out of play so he misses his jump.

FOLLOW THE JUMP-LEADER	This may be performed both indoors and outdoors. Indoor version: the jump-leader stands in one place and continually shifts from one jump-rope exercise to another at will. Those who can not follow are eliminated. The outdoor version: the running jump permits the jump leader to cover any type of terrain that is available, the others following. Those who miss a jump while moving are eliminated.
UPHILL ROPE JUMP	Try this one outdoors in parks, camping or recreational areas on picnics. Select an incline of about 45 degrees. The runoff can be among several as a race, first one to the top. Or the runoff can be individual, according to the fastest time to the hilltop.
SANDSTORM AND SURF SWIRL	Both are beach ropejumps. Both require dexterity and the ability to snap the rope close enough to the surface (in the one instance, on the sand; in the other, the edge of the shoreline) to send up a spray of sand or water *without* interrupting the jump sequence. The highest number of turns is the winner.
JUMP-ROPE SOCCER	This is played with either a soft and light rubber ball or a Ping-Pong ball. The jumpers each attempt to drive the ball to their designated goal entirely with the spin of the rope.
THE WATER CUP	A paper cup is half filled with water and the jumper, seizing it between his teeth, commences jumping *without* spilling the water.

THE
HI-HAT
Another competitive feat. The jumper begins with one hat on his head. The object is to keep the hat from being knocked off. After 20 turns, another hat is added; 20 turns more and another hat. The jumper with the largest number of hats is declared the winner.

FLIP THE
CAP
A bottle-cap is placed on its head and the jumper attempts with the snap of his rope to flip it over. Side bets are in order.

LUCKY
NUMBER
JUMP
The jumper is given a jump limit of 100. Ten jump sets of 10 each. The objective is for the observers to predict the set and number when the jumper's miss will occur. The jumper is not informed of the predicted miss. Side bets can be of several sorts (if the jumper does not miss in his first 100 turns, he repeats): 1. the real luck bonanza of guessing the actual jump number of the miss; 2. the guess of the set number in which the miss is made. The bets are taken on 1st, 2nd, 3rd jump set and so on. (Each set is comprised of 10 jumps, remember?) Or to insure a winner each time, there can be bets taken on the number missed—and whether it is odds or evens.

PARTYTIME
PLOYS
These jump-gems can be used whenever the occasion permits—at house parties, office parties and even private romps if a jumpmate is accessible. What's more, this is your chance to be inventive. Start with this or that jump and take it from there. The one inflexible rule is that the jump rope must

be used. I don't mean to be a killjoy, but that's the kind of book this is.

THE KISS COCKTAIL	The boy or the girl takes up the rope and starts the jump. His opposite jumpmate steps in and, facing the jumper, picks up the same jump beat. Now the heavy exercise begins. The jumpmates must plant ten kisses, lip to lip, without interrupting the rope spin. Smooches on the nose, chin or contact lenses are not pointmakers. A dozen variations of this game are left to the improvisation-minded reader.
THE LEI	All participating jumpers wear the traditional lei as the jumping commences. The object being to unsettle the lei and gradually "climb it" up over the head and toss it free in the act of jumping. Jutting chins, assisting teeth, propping ears are all permitted.
THE PILLION	A Hell's Angels inspiration for hugable hopmates. The "riding position" is taken before the jump begins—the jumper with rope in hand is encircled about the waist from behind by his jumpmate. Don't just stand there! You're supposed to start jumping, remember?
THE JUMP-ROPE ROCK	For the host or hostess who prides himself on novel ideas for group fantasies. The spectacle of what happens to improvised dancing to rock music with a jump rope in hand is something that Fel-

lini would have used for his *Satyricon* if he had thought of it! Wild but kneebuckling laughs guaranteed. To top it all off, you can run a competitive talent show.

JUMP-
ANALYSIS

(Or *J Therapy.*) In our time of body language, or nonverbal behavior, we have come to learn the truth of that old Tin Pan Alley song lyric, "Every little movement has a meaning all its own." And each ropejumper inadvertently exposes his ropejump psyche: bold, tentative, introspective, flirtatious, aspirational or whatever.

So each jump-rope participant, in turn, takes the front-and-center position and begins to jump. This proceeds for intervals of 20 jumps, with each spectator contributing his psychoanalytical reflections. Talk about new forms of encounter therapy—you will never encounter the likes of this one. And for real therapy—you can't beat laughter. The exercise does its bit too!

THE
DOT/DASH-
SPIN

For more Morse than *re*morse, copy out the code on a large pad* so that each person can figure out the message he or she intends to communicate to the others during the respective jump/turn.

The dot/dash message is simple enough to transmit by striking the rope harder on each jump/turn to accent and distinguish the *dash*. A slower turn

```
*A ·– / B –··· / C ··  · / D –·· / E · / F ··–· /
G  ––· / H  ···· / I  ·· / J  ·–·– / K  –·– /
L  ·–·· / M  –– / N  –· / O  ··· / P  ·····  /
Q  ··–· / R  ·–· / S  ··· / T  ––– / U  ··– /
V  ···– / W  ·–– / X  ·–·· / Y  ··–·· / Z  ····–· .
```

gives a space interval. A high jump signals between letters, and *two* high jumps signal between words.

Messages should not exceed five words, and the jumper is to continue to repeat his or her message until the first spectator deciphers it. If all request it, then any word may be repeated. The fact that practically no one knows the code and that all must hastily glance at the board, trying to be the first one to piece together the message, contributes to some hilarious entertainment.

JUMP RHYMES

You can jump as long as you can rhyme. It doesn't matter what words—love, dove, shove, glove, above, and so on—or bits of improvised verse:

> *Must a citizen from the Woodstock Nation*
> *Who has a shabby reputation*
> *In the Nixon Administration*
> *Shabbier with each inflation . . .*

Terrible, yes! And to go from bad to verse with something like:

> *Mini skirts, midi skirts*
> *For all the types of taxi flirts*
> *Fashions foolish, fashions fair,*
> *Mink wiglets, ermine underwear . . .*

And if the meter begins to peter, so much the better, as each jump rhymer desperately grasps at verbal straws, sillier by the moment, as he or she tries to extend the jump count. Talk about putting your foot in your mouth, some of the rhymes that come out spur-of-the-moment are good for laughs all week long.

JUMP
AROUND
THE CLOCK

Get a clock with a sweep-second hand that is plainly visible. Then, one at a time, at the signal GO—and for the period of 60 seconds—each ropejumper takes his turn in trying to get the most jumps per minute. Fun and laughs. If you really want to exhaust your group, try 5 minutes. Whew!

JUMPSTAKES

Everyone participating—and six or more is best —writes a number from 25 to 50 and tosses it into a hat. The hat is shaken and each one makes a choice and begins to jump to that exact number. A miss demands elimination. Each of those who are left—and it could be all the participants—writes a number from 50 to 100 and tosses it into the hat. Choices are made and, once again, jumping and eliminations.

Each time the procedure is repeated, double the jump-count numbers. What do you give your winner? Maybe a week's bedrest! You can begin by putting three prizes—1st, 2nd and 3rd—out where they can be seen. It does wonders for motivation and, besides, the disappointed oohs and ahhs of dropouts add to the fun.

COMPUTER
JUMPMATES

Get one up on the computer matchmaking game. Scramble a roomful of rope-spinning males and females and pair them off according to their matching jump-rope tempos! The eminent scientist

Dr. Grey Walter claims that each of us has a distinct brain rhythm. Some couples may be compatible and others not, according to this. This is not to say that the jump-rope matchup is out to prove anything for science's sake. Not even for goodness' sake!

ASTRO-
JUMPS

In these starry-eyed days of the ascendancy of astrology, almost anything connected with the subject is of interest. Combined with jump-rope activity, the odds are in favor of amusing participation in cozy social groups.

THE ZODIAC
SPIN-OFF

This is a rather intriguing one, and since it depends upon a sound scientific principle, it works surprisingly well. The idea is to have each person, in turn, take up the jump rope and start jumping to the signs of the zodiac. The jumper may recite them for himself, or if unsure of them (everybody knows his own), others may recite them for him or her.

The object is for the spectators to guess the sign of the jumper. Actually, the jumper reveals himself, only he is not aware of it! You see, there is a certain response that will show itself when the individual comes to his own sign.

It is known as the *ideo-motor response,* meaning that the idea or thought causes a muscle reaction. It is what causes the table to move at seances. The spectators won't be aware of exactly how or why they know or guess the jumper's zodiac sign, but they will notice *something.*

Anyway, the jumper continues to jump the zodiac cycle until someone *does* guess it. Usually it happens right off, to the fascination of everyone, jumper *and* spectators! Those true astrology buffs with an eye out for character differences may even be able to guess the jumper's sign from his jump style. At least, they may convince themselves that this is what did it.

Just to have them handy, here are the zodiac signs and character traits attributed to each of them:

ARIES	March 21–April 20	*Pioneer*
TAURUS	April 21–May 20	*Provider*
GEMINI	May 21–June 21	*Versatile*
CANCER	June 22–July 22	*Receiver*
LEO	July 23–August 23	*Ruler*
VIRGO	August 24–September 22	*Perfectionist*
LIBRA	September 23–October 22	*Equalizer*
SCORPIO	October 23–November 22	*Sensual*
SAGITTARIUS	November 23–December 21	*Thinker*
CAPRICORN	December 22–January 20	*Organizer*
AQUARIUS	January 21–February 19	*Altruist*
PISCES	February 20–March 20	*Spiritual*

ASTROJUMP CHARADE   Another jump-rope game using the zodiac character traits calls for ropejumpers to ham it up, exhibiting their best Stanislavsky method. The point is to act out the characteristics of each zodiac sign

—in their jump attitude and style; the mercurial changeability of Gemini, the leadership assertiveness of Leo, and so on. Each jumper, in turn, does his *schtick,* staying with one sign for a maximum of 25 jumps. If the acted-out sign is not guessed, another jumper takes over. The one "listener" is secretly told by each jumper what the sign is as he takes off. So the listener is proof-positive. The "jump star" is the one who completes all of the signs or gets closest to it.

JUMP-ROPE HOROSCOPE MESSAGE

Each participant recites (or has recited for him) the zodiac signs as he takes up his or her jump/turn. He begins with his own sign, which is accepted as dominant, and continues until he makes three misses. The character trait of each sign upon which he misses becomes a subordinate trait. So that, say, a Gemini (versatile) who misses respectively on Scorpio (sensual), Capricorn (organizer) and Pisces (spiritual) may have his message interpreted as: a *versatile* fellow of *sensual* intention whose objective is a *spiritual orgy* (organization).

If you think *that's* awful, wait until you catch some of the wild interpretations of your own group!

CHAPTER 15

COMPETITIVE JUMP-ROPE EVENTS

KARATE HAS ITS brown, black and vari-colored belts to indicate proficiency. Here's the jump-rope rating system:

- *Fleebee* (Novice): uninterrupted jump count of up to 250.
- *Cloudbuster* (Apprentice): uninterrupted jump count of 500 to 1000.
- *Jumpronaut* (Journeyman): uninterrupted jump count of 2000-plus.
- *Space Swami:* uninterrupted jump count of 5000-plus.

Once establishing the jump-rope rating, other competitive events can be run off between those on the same level. There is also the continual incentive for raising the rating to the highest grade. The *Space*

Swami can attempt to establish unsurpassable record-breakers.

The jump-rope-manship qualifier is certain to become popular in offices, campuses and recreational areas. It lends itself to inter-office and intercollegiate competition.

THE JUMP-ROPE RELAY (STATIONARY)	Four jumpers comprise a team, each jumping for a predesignated period. The team with the highest total jump count is the winner. Races may be 4 minutes, 8 minutes or 16 minutes.
THE JUMP-ROPE RELAY	On a track or any open area, with a running distance of 50 yards for each participant. No stick (baton) is passed but a teammate begins running as soon as his predecessor draws abreast of him. Rope must be spun continuously during the run. One miss per runner is permissible, providing the runner stops until he again starts his rope-spin. Running with a "dead" rope or missing more than once is cause for disqualification.
JUMP-ROPE SPRINT	Individual competition. Distances 40 and 60 yards. Same rules as above apply.
THE SLOW-DOWN	An event in which the winner is judged according to the *least* number of jumps during the designated time period. Event can run 1 minute, 2 minutes, 4 minutes.

THE JET SPIN   The most jumps counted during the designated time period. Suggested time: 1 minute, 2 minutes, 4 minutes.

THE EXCEEDER   Competition between two or more jumpers, where each, in turn, tries to exceed the jump total of the other. The runoff is based on a process of elimination.

CHAPTER 16

ENTER—

tHE jumpRoNAuTs

TURN IT OFF/BURN IT OFF! could be the new rallying cry for joyful fitness.

If doing it together is the way of the new world, from bird- to weight-watching, why not . . . *jump-rope*-watching? The "Jumpronauts" has an inspirational ring to it! It would be no problem at all for a group leader—the first one to read this book and pick up the instructions—to organize a group of like-minded people interested in fitness and health. The rallying message—*turn it off/burn it off*—couldn't be more worthwhile and promising.

For the distaff groups in twice-weekly sessions, shapeliness, an alert attractiveness and an improved disposition can be inspiring goals. For male groups, in addition to the goal of an improved appearance, there is that more urgent reason: vigorous cardiovascular exercise to strengthen the heart and release the potentially damaging build-up of daily hypertensions.

The benefits for both sexes have already been adequately covered. And the promise beyond this could be the happy prospect of eating normally again, *sans* diets forever, with a healthy metabolism restored to burn off the excess calories.

The meeting of such Jumpronaut groups would be an exhilarating period of joyful ropejumping, improved exercise proficiency, lots of friendly chatter and the noting of individual progress. This should not be limited to the shedding of pounds and inches, but in renewed energy and vitality and a more affirmative approach to living. No more the dread of so-called exercise workouts, with the emphasis on *work* as a laborious ordeal.

The jump sessions, twice a week, can be loosely arranged into three segments. The free exchange of observations and personal experiences would help to give sharpened insight into those habits and problems confronting the individual in his current lifestyle. It is exceedingly important to become conscious of those factors, which, for each individual, build up tensions, lead to apathy and periods of fatigue and depression, of excessive eating, of emotional frustration.

Then, after the verbal release, would be the general letting-off of steam, a freestyle *jump for joy* as the second segment. The third and final segment would be an organized jump-rope exercise phase, with each individual grading his skills and proficiency and having the benefit of others' rating and suggestions. Each group of 15 should have a jumpronaut leader and assistant.

Jumpronaut groups can arrange their jump-rope activity to coincide with other events such as bowling, mah-jongg and various hobby and club meetings. For sunny days, outdoor meetings could be arranged in convenient places like public parks and on country-club or other convenient grounds.

The movement is certain to travel fast with exposure. Few activities are as contagious as that of ropejumping. And for those with a crusading spirit, there are few involvements that can be as satisfying as the communication of a physical-fitness movement for the promotion of healthier, more joyous and longer lives. Furthermore, it is an activity that can be promoted at every level, for all age groups. Jumpronauts will find easy recruits to the idea of "having fun with fitness."

PART IV THE JUMP-ROPE

PERSONALIZER

CHAPTER 17 **THE ENERGY/ RHYTHM PROFILE**

No SYSTEM, whether for diet or exercise, can be exactly right for everyone. Some of the individual differences which should be taken into account are:

- *Metabolism* The rate at which the body uses food for energy, repair and maintenance.
- *Performance Rhythms* We all have performance rates at which we function best. More natural pacing means improved performance with less stress to the system.

- *Body Types* Medical science classifies three basic somatotypes:

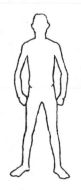 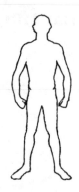 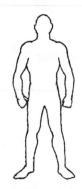

Ectomorphic
(small frame)

Endomorphic
(medium frame)

Mesomorphic
(large frame)

Though we may combine some characteristics of more than one, we all are generally classifiable as one of these types. Because of the differences in body structure, we may require more of one type of exercise than another or more or less exercise generally.

- *Activity Schedules* The personal differences in our lives: sex, marital status, age, occupational differences, psychological attitudes—all are determinants of how much activity and the type of activity we are involved in and how much we require.

The objective in this section is to help you pinpoint many of these personal variations. Naturally, we shall have to make approximations and use certain accepted standards. But suggestions will be included to enable you to modify and shape the exercise system to apply more personally to your individual differences.

CHAPTER 18 **YOUR E.Q.**

(ENERGY QUOTIENT)

SOME IMPORTANT questions about ourselves that few of us know the answers to are:

- How much energy do you use up each day?
- How much food do you require to maintain that energy level?
- How much is excess and thus deposited as fatty tissue?
- How much physical activity are you actually getting?

If we could answer these questions about ourselves, we would be in a better position to adjust and balance: FOOD INTAKE/ENERGY OUTPUT

Isn't it surprising that most people are vague about this most crucial balance for good health and physical fitness? Consider the term—"calorie." It represents the unpleasant weight-gaining measure of each unit of food. That is a far cry from its original meaning: "CALORIE: *the measure of energy produced by food.*" It is strictly an energy rating.

Every movement and bodily process represent a discharge of energy. Each has a calorie measure. For example, the energy required to write a letter: if it takes you twenty minutes, it costs you approximately 30 calories! The action of raising a hand to your mouth to puff a cigarette requires an energy output. Even the jaw-chewing and swallowing actions in eating do. If a meal takes you half an hour, it costs you 12½ calories.

The measure for food requirement is the quota of physical activity. But this concept has been blurred in our society of great abundance and limited physical activity. We began to eat rich and tasty foods without any thought of the physical work we have had to produce. Food intake has lost its direct relationship to energy output.

Now, food intake and energy output are commonly divided into two separate elements. When out of balance with each other, they are the major health hazards of our times.

Excessive food intake results in the condition of "overweight" (obesity), for which we consider the solution to be *dieting*.

Insufficient energy output is the result of "underwork" and a poorly conditioned body, for which we consider the solution to be *physical-fitness exercises*.

We are all familiar with the *calorie value* of common foods. The list that follows presents the other half of the coin—*the calorie cost of common activities*. It has a twofold purpose: 1. to reunite, in the reader's mind, food intake and energy output as inseparable parts of one energy process. This will make you more aware of the calorie value of food consumed as against the calorie cost of activities engaged in; and, 2., to enable you to arrive at a personal energy measure of your own activities. This will give you a more accurate picture of the amount of exercise that your body requires.

DAILY ACTIVITY ENERGY OUTPUT

How the Listing That Follows Is Arranged: it deals with the energy output in a typical 24-hour day.

Column I lists the day's activities from waking, arising, washing, dressing, transportation to a job, the working day, eating meals, the evening's relaxation and the night's sleep. All are itemized in the general order in which they are performed. The work is distinguished according to medium-heavy work, medium work, light work.

Column II establishes the energy measure for each activity (calories per hour).

Column III estimates the approximate time spent performing each activity.

Column IV represents the total daily cost in calories for each activity.

I. ACTIVITY	II. CALORIE MEASURE PER HR.	III. ACTIVITY PERIOD	IV. ACTUAL CALORIE COST
Eating	25	30 minutes (breakfast)	10
		1 hour (lunch)	25
Grooming	100	10 minutes (morning)	15
Dressing	125	15–20 minutes (morning)	50
Walking	200	10 minutes (morning preparations)	20
Driving	75	45 minutes	55
WORKING DAY			
Moderately active manual labor	275	8 hours	2200
Moderately active housewife*			1400
Office work	150	8 hours	1200
Driving	75	45 minutes (evening transportation)	55
Walking	200	10 minutes (evening transportation)	20
Eating	25	1 hour (dinner)	25
TV-Watching	80	2 hours	160
Sleeping	75	8 hours	600

To arrive at total, select the level from the Working Day section closest to your own and add Column IV for energy cost per day.

* The housewife's day was divided as follows: 4 hours of housework at 250 calories per hour. One hour of walking, perhaps for keeping the youngsters in tow or serving meals, at a calorie cost of 200. One hour of shopping at a calorie cost of 200.

YOUR
PERSONAL
ENERGY
RATING

Here is how you can make the adjustments to arrive at a closer picture of the extent and kind of
your daily activity:

- Use the Daily Energy-Output Diary on p.
  118. Fill in your activities daily, for any
  typical week. Note the time you spend doing
  them.
- Refer to the list below for the energy rating
  of the various activities. (In instances where
  some may be absent, you will be able to
  equate them with activities generally re-
  quiring similar levels of effort).

ACTIVITY	CALORIE COST PER HOUR
Eating	25
Grooming	100
Dressing	125
Walking	200
Driving	75
TV-Watching	80
Sleeping	75
Golf	300
Bowling	350–400
Dancing (relaxed to high-activity)	250–500
Piano-Playing	75–125
Walking (vigorously)	300
Swimming (moderate crawl)	600
Standing	100–150
Sitting	100
Writing	100
Typewriting	130–160
Singing	125

The Daily
Energy-
Output
Diary

MONDAY

Type of Activity	Amount of Time	Calorie Cost
_____	_____	_____
_____	_____	_____
_____	_____	_____
_____	_____	_____
_____	_____	_____
_____	_____	_____
_____	_____	_____
_____	_____	_____
_____	_____	_____
_____	_____	_____

TOTAL: _____

THE DAILY   TUESDAY
ENERGY-
OUTPUT   Amount   Calorie
DIARY   Type of Activity   of Time   Cost

Type of Activity	Amount of Time	Calorie Cost
_____	____	____
_____	____	____
_____	____	____
_____	____	____
_____	____	____
_____	____	____
_____	____	____
_____	____	____
_____	____	____
_____	____	____

TOTAL: _____

THE DAILY ENERGY-OUTPUT DIARY	WEDNESDAY		
	Type of Activity	Amount of Time	Calorie Cost
	_____	_____	_____
	_____	_____	_____
	_____	_____	_____
	_____	_____	_____
	_____	_____	_____
	_____	_____	_____
	_____	_____	_____
	_____	_____	_____
	_____	_____	_____
	_____	_____	_____
		TOTAL:	_____

THE DAILY **THURSDAY**
ENERGY-
OUTPUT   Amount   Calorie
  DIARY Type of Activity   of Time Cost

_____ _____ _____

_____ _____ _____

_____ _____ _____

_____ _____ _____

_____ _____ _____

_____ _____ _____

_____ _____ _____

_____ _____ _____

_____ _____ _____

_____ _____ _____

TOTAL: _____

THE DAILY ENERGY-OUTPUT DIARY	FRIDAY Type of Activity	Amount of Time	Calorie Cost
	_____	_____	_____
	_____	_____	_____
	_____	_____	_____
	_____	_____	_____
	_____	_____	_____
	_____	_____	_____
	_____	_____	_____
	_____	_____	_____
	_____	_____	_____
	_____	_____	_____
		TOTAL:	_____

THE DAILY SATURDAY
ENERGY-
OUTPUT   Amount   Calorie
DIARY   Type of Activity   of Time   Cost

Type of Activity	Amount of Time	Calorie Cost
_____	____	____
_____	____	____
_____	____	____
_____	____	____
_____	____	____
_____	____	____
_____	____	____
_____	____	____
_____	____	____
_____	____	____

TOTAL: _____

THE DAILY ENERGY-OUTPUT DIARY	SUNDAY		
	Type of Activity	Amount of Time	Calorie Cost
	_____	_____	_____
	_____	_____	_____
	_____	_____	_____
	_____	_____	_____
	_____	_____	_____
	_____	_____	_____
	_____	_____	_____
	_____	_____	_____
	_____	_____	_____
	_____	_____	_____
		TOTAL:	_____

CHAPTER 19 pERSONAl RhyThM

pATTERNS

Dr. Hans Selye of the Institute of Experimental
Medicine at the University of Montreal has been
able to prove with his research that we each have
work cycles at which we perform best. There are
regular times when our energy levels are low and
others when they are at a peak. He has explained
that each person has a personal fatigue pattern.
What's more, it is possible to identify this personal rhythm and to gear our efforts accordingly.

For example, if we know our peak energy is at
10:00 A.M. and at 3:00 P.M., we would do well
to handle our important and more difficult tasks at
these hours. If we begin to coast at 11:00 A.M. or
peter out at 4:00 P.M., this might be the ideal time
to take a coffeebreak or forty winks, if it is possible.
This personal pacing may reveal hunger patterns
for some readers of which they were not aware.
We might do better to shift our mealtimes accord-

ingly. Sleep patterns can be reexamined for that matter. Many of us are tired because we *oversleep!* We may sleep more or less than our systems require. A knowledge of your personal daily performance rhythms will point out the best time of the day for you to take exercise.

YOUR DAILY RHYTHM DIARY *

You can track your daily rhythms on the chart that follows. It will help you to answer such questions as:

- At what time or times during the day do you feel a letdown, or tired and sleepy?
- At what time or times do you feel the most energetic and get the most accomplished?

These questions have to do not only with performance but also with feelings of brightness, optimism or animation, compared to less exuberant periods.

* If you choose, you can complete *both* your Daily Energy-Output Diary and Personal Rhythm Diary during the same period.

DAILY   MONDAY   Energy Level (check one):
RHYTHM   High   Medium   Low
DIARY   A.M.   7:00   _____   _____   _____
                7:30   _____   _____   _____
                8:00   _____   _____   _____
                8:30   _____   _____   _____
                9:00   _____   _____   _____
                9:30   _____   _____   _____
                10:00   _____   _____   _____
                10:30   _____   _____   _____
                11:00   _____   _____   _____
                11:30   _____   _____   _____
                Noon   _____   _____   _____
        P.M.   12:30   _____   _____   _____
                1:00   _____   _____   _____
                1:30   _____   _____   _____
                2:00   _____   _____   _____
                2:30   _____   _____   _____
                3:00   _____   _____   _____
                3:30   _____   _____   _____
                4:00   _____   _____   _____
                4:30   _____   _____   _____
                5:00   _____   _____   _____
                5:30   _____   _____   _____
                6:00   _____   _____   _____
                6:30   _____   _____   _____
                7:00   _____   _____   _____
                7:30   _____   _____   _____
                8:00   _____   _____   _____
                8:30   _____   _____   _____
                9:00   _____   _____   _____
                9:30   _____   _____   _____
                10:00   _____   _____   _____
                10:30   _____   _____   _____
                11:00   _____   _____   _____
                11:30   _____   _____   _____
                Midnight _____   _____   _____

SPECIAL   Note instances
COMMENTS   when you're in   _____
            particular good
            humor, or feeling   _____
            confident or tired
            and dejected.   _____

DAILY RHYTHM DIARY	TUESDAY		Energy Level (check one): High Medium Low		
	A.M.	7:00	_____	_____	_____
		7:30	_____	_____	_____
		8:00	_____	_____	_____
		8:30	_____	_____	_____
		9:00	_____	_____	_____
		9:30	_____	_____	_____
		10:00	_____	_____	_____
		10:30	_____	_____	_____
		11:00	_____	_____	_____
		11:30	_____	_____	_____
		Noon	_____	_____	_____
	P.M.	12:30	_____	_____	_____
		1:00	_____	_____	_____
		1:30	_____	_____	_____
		2:00	_____	_____	_____
		2:30	_____	_____	_____
		3:00	_____	_____	_____
		3:30	_____	_____	_____
		4:00	_____	_____	_____
		4:30	_____	_____	_____
		5:00	_____	_____	_____
		5:30	_____	_____	_____
		6:00	_____	_____	_____
		6:30	_____	_____	_____
		7:00	_____	_____	_____
		7:30	_____	_____	_____
		8:00	_____	_____	_____
		8:30	_____	_____	_____
		9:00	_____	_____	_____
		9:30	_____	_____	_____
		10:00	_____	_____	_____
		10:30	_____	_____	_____
		11:00	_____	_____	_____
		11:30	_____	_____	_____
		Midnight	_____	_____	_____

SPECIAL
COMMENTS

Note instances
when you're in
particular good
humor, or feeling
confident or tired
and dejected.

_____

_____

_____

DAILY RHYTHM DIARY	WEDNESDAY		Energy Level (check one):		
			High	Medium	Low
	A.M.	7:00	_____	_____	_____
		7:30	_____	_____	_____
		8:00	_____	_____	_____
		8:30	_____	_____	_____
		9:00	_____	_____	_____
		9:30	_____	_____	_____
		10:00	_____	_____	_____
		10:30	_____	_____	_____
		11:00	_____	_____	_____
		11:30	_____	_____	_____
		Noon	_____	_____	_____
	P.M.	12:30	_____	_____	_____
		1:00	_____	_____	_____
		1:30	_____	_____	_____
		2:00	_____	_____	_____
		2:30	_____	_____	_____
		3:00	_____	_____	_____
		3:30	_____	_____	_____
		4:00	_____	_____	_____
		4:30	_____	_____	_____
		5:00	_____	_____	_____
		5:30	_____	_____	_____
		6:00	_____	_____	_____
		6:30	_____	_____	_____
		7:00	_____	_____	_____
		7:30	_____	_____	_____
		8:00	_____	_____	_____
		8:30	_____	_____	_____
		9:00	_____	_____	_____
		9:30	_____	_____	_____
		10:00	_____	_____	_____
		10:30	_____	_____	_____
		11:00	_____	_____	_____
		11:30	_____	_____	_____
		Midnight	_____	_____	_____

SPECIAL COMMENTS

Note instances when you're in particular good humor, or feeling confident or tired and dejected.

_____

_____

_____

DAILY	THURSDAY		Energy Level (check one):		
RHYTHM			High	Medium	Low
DIARY	A.M.	7:00	_____	_____	_____
		7:30	_____	_____	_____
		8:00	_____	_____	_____
		8:30	_____	_____	_____
		9:00	_____	_____	_____
		9:30	_____	_____	_____
		10:00	_____	_____	_____
		10:30	_____	_____	_____
		11:00	_____	_____	_____
		11:30	_____	_____	_____
		Noon	_____	_____	_____
	P.M.	12:30	_____	_____	_____
		1:00	_____	_____	_____
		1:30	_____	_____	_____
		2:00	_____	_____	_____
		2:30	_____	_____	_____
		3:00	_____	_____	_____
		3:30	_____	_____	_____
		4:00	_____	_____	_____
		4:30	_____	_____	_____
		5:00	_____	_____	_____
		5:30	_____	_____	_____
		6:00	_____	_____	_____
		6:30	_____	_____	_____
		7:00	_____	_____	_____
		7:30	_____	_____	_____
		8:00	_____	_____	_____
		8:30	_____	_____	_____
		9:00	_____	_____	_____
		9:30	_____	_____	_____
		10:00	_____	_____	_____
		10:30	_____	_____	_____
		11:00	_____	_____	_____
		11:30	_____	_____	_____
		Midnight	_____	_____	_____

SPECIAL
COMMENTS

Note instances when you're in particular good humor, or feeling confident or tired and dejected.

_____

_____

_____

DAILY RHYTHM DIARY	FRIDAY		Energy Level (check one):		
			High	Medium	Low
A.M.		7:00	_____	_____	_____
		7:30	_____	_____	_____
		8:00	_____	_____	_____
		8:30	_____	_____	_____
		9:00	_____	_____	_____
		9:30	_____	_____	_____
		10:00	_____	_____	_____
		10:30	_____	_____	_____
		11:00	_____	_____	_____
		11:30	_____	_____	_____
		Noon	_____	_____	_____
P.M.		12:30	_____	_____	_____
		1:00	_____	_____	_____
		1:30	_____	_____	_____
		2:00	_____	_____	_____
		2:30	_____	_____	_____
		3:00	_____	_____	_____
		3:30	_____	_____	_____
		4:00	_____	_____	_____
		4:30	_____	_____	_____
		5:00	_____	_____	_____
		5:30	_____	_____	_____
		6:00	_____	_____	_____
		6:30	_____	_____	_____
		7:00	_____	_____	_____
		7:30	_____	_____	_____
		8:00	_____	_____	_____
		8:30	_____	_____	_____
		9:00	_____	_____	_____
		9:30	_____	_____	_____
		10:00	_____	_____	_____
		10:30	_____	_____	_____
		11:00	_____	_____	_____
		11:30	_____	_____	_____
		Midnight	_____	_____	_____

SPECIAL COMMENTS   Note instances when you're in particular good humor, or feeling confident or tired and dejected.

_____

_____

_____

DAILY RHYTHM DIARY	SATURDAY		Energy Level (check one):		
			High	Medium	Low
A.M.		7:00	_____	_____	_____
		7:30	_____	_____	_____
		8:00	_____	_____	_____
		8:30	_____	_____	_____
		9:00	_____	_____	_____
		9:30	_____	_____	_____
		10:00	_____	_____	_____
		10:30	_____	_____	_____
		11:00	_____	_____	_____
		11:30	_____	_____	_____
		Noon	_____	_____	_____
P.M.		12:30	_____	_____	_____
		1:00	_____	_____	_____
		1:30	_____	_____	_____
		2:00	_____	_____	_____
		2:30	_____	_____	_____
		3:00	_____	_____	_____
		3:30	_____	_____	_____
		4:00	_____	_____	_____
		4:30	_____	_____	_____
		5:00	_____	_____	_____
		5:30	_____	_____	_____
		6:00	_____	_____	_____
		6:30	_____	_____	_____
		7:00	_____	_____	_____
		7:30	_____	_____	_____
		8:00	_____	_____	_____
		8:30	_____	_____	_____
		9:00	_____	_____	_____
		9:30	_____	_____	_____
		10:00	_____	_____	_____
		10:30	_____	_____	_____
		11:00	_____	_____	_____
		11:30	_____	_____	_____
		Midnight	_____	_____	_____

SPECIAL COMMENTS Note instances when you're in particular good humor, or feeling confident or tired and dejected.

_____

_____

_____

DAILY RHYTHM DIARY	SUNDAY		Energy Level (check one):		
			High	Medium	Low
A.M.		7:00	___	___	___
		7:30	___	___	___
		8:00	___	___	___
		8:30	___	___	___
		9:00	___	___	___
		9:30	___	___	___
		10:00	___	___	___
		10:30	___	___	___
		11:00	___	___	___
		11:30	___	___	___
		Noon	___	___	___
P.M.		12:30	___	___	___
		1:00	___	___	___
		1:30	___	___	___
		2:00	___	___	___
		2:30	___	___	___
		3:00	___	___	___
		3:30	___	___	___
		4:00	___	___	___
		4:30	___	___	___
		5:00	___	___	___
		5:30	___	___	___
		6:00	___	___	___
		6:30	___	___	___
		7:00	___	___	___
		7:30	___	___	___
		8:00	___	___	___
		8:30	___	___	___
		9:00	___	___	___
		9:30	___	___	___
		10:00	___	___	___
		10:30	___	___	___
		11:00	___	___	___
		11:30	___	___	___
		Midnight	___	___	___

SPECIAL COMMENTS   Note instances when you're in particular good humor, or feeling confident or tired and dejected.

_____

_____

_____

PERSONAL-
IZING THE
JUMP-ROPE
EXERCISE

Here is where we begin to apply the special focus of the different jump-rope exercises. As previously explained, all of the exercises have general conditioning and circulatory benefits. But the changes in body position focus special stress upon particular body areas. Here's how to use this section and the list following:

- Check off in *List I* the physical-fitness problems to which you would like to lend special emphasis.
- Choose from *List II* the jump-rope exercises that concentrate more fully upon your special physical-fitness problems. They are identified by matching letters.
- Use them to replace others in your regular jump-rope exercise sequences.

LIST I   *I need to:*

A   relieve my body of tension and stress.

B   overcome shortness of breath and develop endurance.

C   develop my stomach muscles.

D   firm up my underarms.

E   stretch my neckline and face muscles.

F   get rid of back stiffness.

G   trim down my buttocks.

H   develop hip flexibility.

I   stimulate pelvic movements.

J trim down my thighs.

K strengthen my knees.

L strengthen my ankles.

M get rid of foot ache.

N firm up general flabbiness.

O improve my coordination.

LIST II All jump-rope exercises are circulatory and general conditioners. You need not be concerned about repeating one or several special exercises to the exclusion of others of the regular jump-rope exercise sequences.

A THE SAG
   For muscle stiffness; releases nervous tension.

B THE PEACOCK
   Develops more complete respiration.

B THE MARATHON
   Builds endurance.

C THE GREYHOUND
   Builds and strengthens abdominal muscle wall.

D THE WIDE WING
   Arms and torso conditioner.

E THE STAR-SWALLOW
   Encourages firmer and more youthful jaw and neckline.

F THE SWAYBACK
   Strengthens tendons of back and spinal column.

F, K   THE GROUCHO
Conditions lower back and knee joints.

F, H   THE HIP SWING
Prevents stiffening of hip joints, lower spinal column.

F, H, I   THE ELEVATOR
Hip-girdle, pelvis and small-of-back conditioner.

G, H   HOP 'N' JUMP
Thigh and buttock conditioner.

G, H, I   THE PRANCE
Pelvis strengthener; thigh and buttock conditioner.

G, I, J   THE SPACE MAN
High-level developer of large thigh and buttock muscles; pelvic conditioner.

H, I   THE KANGAROO
Intense hip-girdle and pelvis conditioner.

H, K, L   THE PIGEON-TOE
Strengthens ankle, knee and hip joints.

I, J   THE CHAPLIN
Benefits inner thighs and pelvis; outer buttocks.

L, M   THE TOE JUMP
Powerful developer of feet and ankles, leg muscles.

N   THE STIFF
Head-to-toe muscle and joint conditioner.

O   THE DOUBLE-SPIN
Builds high-level muscle coordination.

O   THE CRISS-CROSS
Improves timing and high-level coordination.

THE OFFICE
JUMP-WEEK
SCHEDULE

While there are those who prefer going at exercise as impulse commands, others perform more effectively with a more organized plan (See p. 138). This can have its benefits, as well. For example, you may wish to gear your jump-rope exercise to burn off energy according to the level of your daily office schedule, in which case you can figure this out in the Daily Energy-Output Diary (p. 118). With a general energy rating for the Jump-Rope Activity (p. 117), your next step can be to determine how much jump-rope exercise you will require; and then, which exercises they should be. This last will be determined by the level of your jump-rope proficiency.

If you know pretty well when and at which times in your work schedule, and even *where* in your office, you can manage some daily ropejumping, such planning is relatively simple. You may wish, as well, to work in special emphasis on your thighs or back or whatever your individual figure or physique requirements are. Reference to *Personalizing the Jump-Rope Exercise* on p. 134 will help you in this. At this point, you will be able to set up your office jump-rope exercise for the week, with variations for novelty's sake, if you choose, from day to day.

For those who happen to favor this method: determine your physical activity and body conditioning needs. Jot them down by name under each day of the week in the Office Jump-Week Schedule and the jump/turn number under the *count* column. *Rate* yourself on your exercise performance: A = excellent; B = good; C = fair; D = poor. Observe your rate of improvement. Tuck the schedule into the corner of your desk blotter or tape it to the wall, under the calendar, if you want to keep your activity from becoming a group-participation event.

OFFICE JUMP-WEEK SCHEDULE	Week of _____ *(date)* Exercise	Exercise Period _____ *(time of day)* Count	Rate
Monday	_____	_____	_____
	_____	_____	_____
	_____	_____	_____
	_____	_____	_____
Tuesday	_____	_____	_____
	_____	_____	_____
	_____	_____	_____
Wednesday	_____	_____	_____
	_____	_____	_____
	_____	_____	_____
Thursday	_____	_____	_____
	_____	_____	_____
	_____	_____	_____
	_____	_____	_____
Friday	_____	_____	_____
	_____	_____	_____
	_____	_____	_____
	_____	_____	_____

REFERENCES

Books that have furnished the author with valuable reference material include:

The Vital Balance, Karl Menninger, M.D.; New York: Viking Press, 1963.

The Wisdom of the Body, W. B. Cannon; New York: Norton, 1932.

On Aggression, Konrad Lorenz; New York: Harcourt, Brace & World, Inc., 1966.

Rhythmic Activity in Animal Physiology and Behavior, J. Cloudsley-Thompson; New York: Academic Press, 1961.

Jogging, Aerobics and Diet, Roy Ald; New York: New American Library, 1968.

Human Sexual Inadequacy, William H. Masters and Virginia E. Johnson; Boston: Little Brown & Company, 1970.

About the Author

A Whitemanesque poet at the age of seventeen, Roy Ald went to work with a traveling carnival, wrote and published a children's magazine, and wrote and sold a body development course. An equally versatile adult, Mr. Ald is a prize-winning poet, a writer on many subjects, including sociology and fiction, and, most prominently, a physical fitness authority. He has conducted physical fitness courses, lectures, and demonstrations for groups across the country. His current books in the field in addition to *Jump for Joy!*, are *Physical Fitness after 35, Cycling,* and *Jogging, Aerobics, & Diet.*

72-01003